The NEURODIVERGENT COOKBOOK

Easy Sensory-Friendly Meals Designed for Picky Eaters, ARFID, OCD, ADHD, and Autistic Children and Adults

by Mary Wojcik

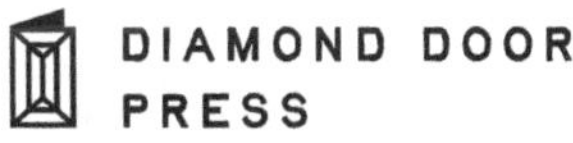

DIAMOND DOOR PRESS

This is a work of nonfiction. All recipes contained in this book are original creations by the author and are not intended to copy or infringe upon any existing recipes. Any resemblance to other recipes is coincidental.

While every effort has been made to ensure accuracy, the information in this book is provided "as is," without warranty of any kind, express or implied. The publisher and author disclaim any liability arising directly or indirectly from the use or application of any information contained herein. Readers should exercise their own judgment and, where appropriate, consult a qualified professional (including a physician, dietitian, or nutritionist) before acting on any information provided.

Published by
Diamond Door Press
New York, NY

Printed in the United States of America

First Edition

ISBN: 978-1-971159-00-3

diamonddoorpress.com

To all the neurodivergent adults and children who deserve food that feels safe, comforting, and full of love. This book is for you.

TABLE OF CONTENTS

INTRODUCTION 7

CHAPTER 1: Creating Your Personal Safe Food List 11

CHAPTER 2: Kitchen Setup for Success 15

CHAPTER 3: Smooth Smoothies and Juices 21

Perfect Vanilla Smoothie 22
Chocolate Peanut Butter Power Smoothie 25
Peach Banana Classic Smoothie 26
Anti-Anxiety Pineapple Smoothie with Chamomile Tea 29
Room Temperature Fruit Juice 30
Liquid Meal Replacement Smoothie 31
Freeze-Ahead Fruit Smoothie Packs 33
Green Juice That Doesn't Taste Green 34

CHAPTER 4: It's All About the Chicken 37

Perfect Breaded Chicken Tenders 38
Crispy Baked Chicken Nuggets 41
Plain Poached Chicken Breast 42
Grilled Chicken Strips 45
Panko Breaded Chicken Drumsticks 46
Slow Cooker Shredded Chicken 49
Ground Chicken Patties 50
Chicken Meatballs 51
Broiled Chicken Thighs 53
Barbecue Baked Chicken Wings 54

CHAPTER 5: Comfort Foods & Sweet Regulation 57

Go-To Hamburger 59
Perfect Buttered Pasta 60
Ultimate White Rice 63
Cinnamon Sugar Toast 64
No Lumps Mashed Potatoes 66
French Toast Sticks 67
Classic Grilled Cheese 69
Baked Mac and Cheese 70
Simple Pancakes 73
Soft Chocolate Chip Cookies 74

CHAPTER 6: 15 Minutes or Less 77

3-Minute Microwave Scrambled Eggs 78
5-Minute Cheese Quesadilla 81
Instant Oatmeal Upgrade Bowl 82
Avocado Toast 85
Quick Teriyaki Tuna Rice Bowl 86
Microwaved Loaded Baked Potato 87
Emergency Snack Plate with Baguette 89
Shutdown Day Survival Meal 90

CHAPTER 7: Sensory Considerate Foods 93

Perfectly Crispy Roasted Potato Wedges 94
Extra Smooth Tomato Soup 97
Crunchy Pita Chips with Extra Smooth Hummus 98
Crunchy Coconut Shrimp 100
Crunchy Cashew Chicken and Rice 102
Room Temperature Creamy Pasta Salad 105
Crisp Cinnamon Sugar Pita Chips 106
Silky Sweet Vanilla Yogurt Dip 107
Chewy Oatmeal Cookies 109
Super Smooth Banana “Ice Cream” 110

CHAPTER 8: Safe Food Transformations 113

Butternut Squash Mac and Cheese 114
Pizza with Cauliflower Crust 117
Plain Pasta with Hidden Veggie Sauce 118
Veggie-Packed Meatballs 119
Zucchini Chocolate Muffins 121
Sweet Potato Pancakes 122
Hidden Veggie Brownies 125
Secretly Nutritious Cookies 126

CHAPTER 9: Executive Function Friendly 129

Easy Sheet Pan Cheesy Nachos 130
Wrap and Roll Lunch 133
Sheet Pan Chicken and Vegetables 134
One-Pot Creamy Pasta 135
Throw-and-Go Slow Cooker Beef Stew 137
Snack Plate Dinner 138
Baked Pasta Casserole 141
Freezer Breakfast Egg Muffins 142

CHAPTER 10: ARFID-Focused Solutions 145

Concentrated Nutrition Drink 146
High-Energy Snack Balls with Chocolate Sauce 149
High-Calorie Cheese Sauce 150
Calorie-Dense Pasta 151
Energy-Dense Muffins 153
Liquid Meal Soup 154
Calorie-Packed Toast 157
Protein-Packed Pancakes 158

CHAPTER 11: Food Chaining Adventures 161

Food Chaining Ideas 162

INDEX 164

ABOUT THE AUTHOR 166

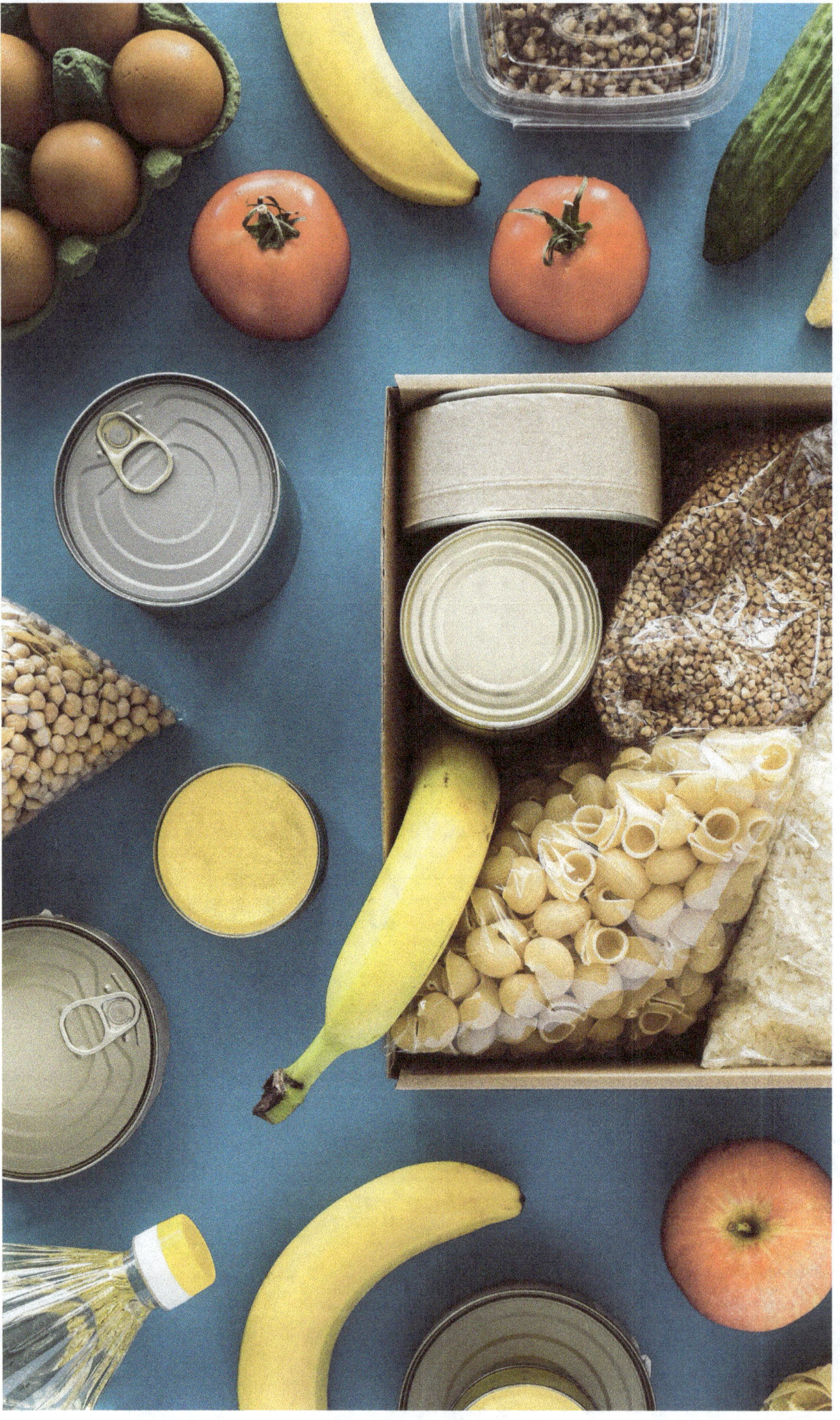

INTRODUCTION: UNDERSTANDING NEURODIVERGENT EATING

Food doesn't have to be a battle, but sometimes it feels like one. If you're neurodivergent, or if you're a parent trying to nourish a neurodivergent child, you know that eating involves so much more than just being hungry. Maybe you have textures that make you cringe, smells that overwhelm you, or a handful of trusted foods that keep you going when everything else feels like too much. Maybe you're watching your child struggle with the same challenges. You're doing your best, and that matters.

If anyone has ever made you feel bad about being "picky" or told you to "just get over it," this book sees you. Your relationship with food is valid exactly as it is. Your sensory experiences are real, your safe foods are important, and you deserve to eat in a way that feels good for your body and your brain.

This cookbook isn't about convincing you to eat differently. It's about meeting you where you are and giving you tools that actually work, whether you're cooking for yourself or for someone you love. Some recipes will feel familiar and comforting. Others might gently expand what's possible when you're ready. But everything here is designed with understanding, not judgment. Because everyone should feel nourished and supported, exactly as you are.

What Makes Eating Different for Neurodivergent Individuals

For people with Autism, OCD (Obsessive-Compulsive Disorder), ADHD (Attention Deficit Hyperactivity Disorder), ARFID (Avoidant/Restrictive Food Intake Disorder) and the like, eating can be about much more than taste.

Sensory processing can shape food acceptance. A certain texture, smell, or visual presentation can make or break a meal.

Predictability helps reduce anxiety. Safe foods, those familiar, reliable options you know will be consistent every time, can be an anchor in an otherwise unpredictable day.

Energy demands from planning, cooking, and cleaning can be significant. Even a simple recipe can feel like a big task on a low-energy day.

Safe Foods as a Foundation

Safe foods are not "bad" foods or something to outgrow. They are essential tools for regulation, comfort, and nourishment. They create stability, especially during times of sensory overload, stress, or burnout. This book builds from that foundation rather than asking you to abandon it. You will see recipes that honor safe foods as they are, along with gentle variations for when you are curious about something new.

The Sensory Science of Eating

Texture, temperature, and appearance often matter as much as, or more than, taste. Smooth, uniform foods can be calming. Crunchy foods can provide grounding and predictable feedback. Mixed or inconsistent textures may be more difficult to manage. That is why every recipe in this book includes **Texture** and **Sensory Notes** so there are no surprises.

Executive Function and Meal Planning

Cooking is more than just following a recipe. It involves decision-making, gathering ingredients, timing steps, and cleaning up afterward. On days when your mental load is already heavy, that can be too much. This book includes low-energy ("low-spoon") options, no-cook ideas, batch-prep strategies, and "emergency" meals for days when you need something fast and familiar.

Food Chaining: Gentle Expansion

Food chaining is a slow, low-pressure way to build variety into your diet. By starting with something familiar and making a tiny change, a new coating on chicken tenders, a drop of olive oil on plain pasta, or a microscopic addition of a new ingredient, you or your child can explore without feeling pushed. *Chapter 11: Food Chaining Adventures* walks you through step-by-step bridge recipes to guide this process.

Supporting Families and Reducing Conflict

Mealtimes can become a source of tension in families, especially when eating preferences differ. This cookbook can help bridge that gap by offering recipes and strategies that respect neurodivergent needs while still providing balanced, satisfying meals for everyone at the table.

How to Use This Cookbook

Each recipe includes information to help you quickly decide if it fits your current energy and comfort level:

Spoon Rating

Based on "Spoon Theory," which uses spoons as a symbol for daily energy reserves. One spoon means minimal effort. Five spoons means more steps and more time.

Serving Size

Tells how many servings each recipe makes

Texture

Describes the primary texture: smooth, crunchy, chewy, or soft.

Temperature

Lists whether the recipe is best served warm, cold, or at room temperature.

Prep Time

An estimate of how long the recipe will take from start to finish.

Calories per Serving

An approximate number for those who want nutritional guidance.

Sensory Notes

Extra details about smell, mouthfeel, or visual elements that might matter for acceptance.

Spoon Rating: ⅠⅠⅠⅠ
Makes: 3–4 servings
Texture: Crunchy outside, tender inside
Temperature: Hot
Prep Time: 20 minutes
Calories per serving: ~300–350
Sensory Notes: Mild flavor, small manageable pieces, consistent texture

Use these details to match the recipe to your needs in the moment. Some days you might be open to trying something new. Other days you might stick with the most familiar options. Both are valid. This book is here to make those choices easier and more supportive.

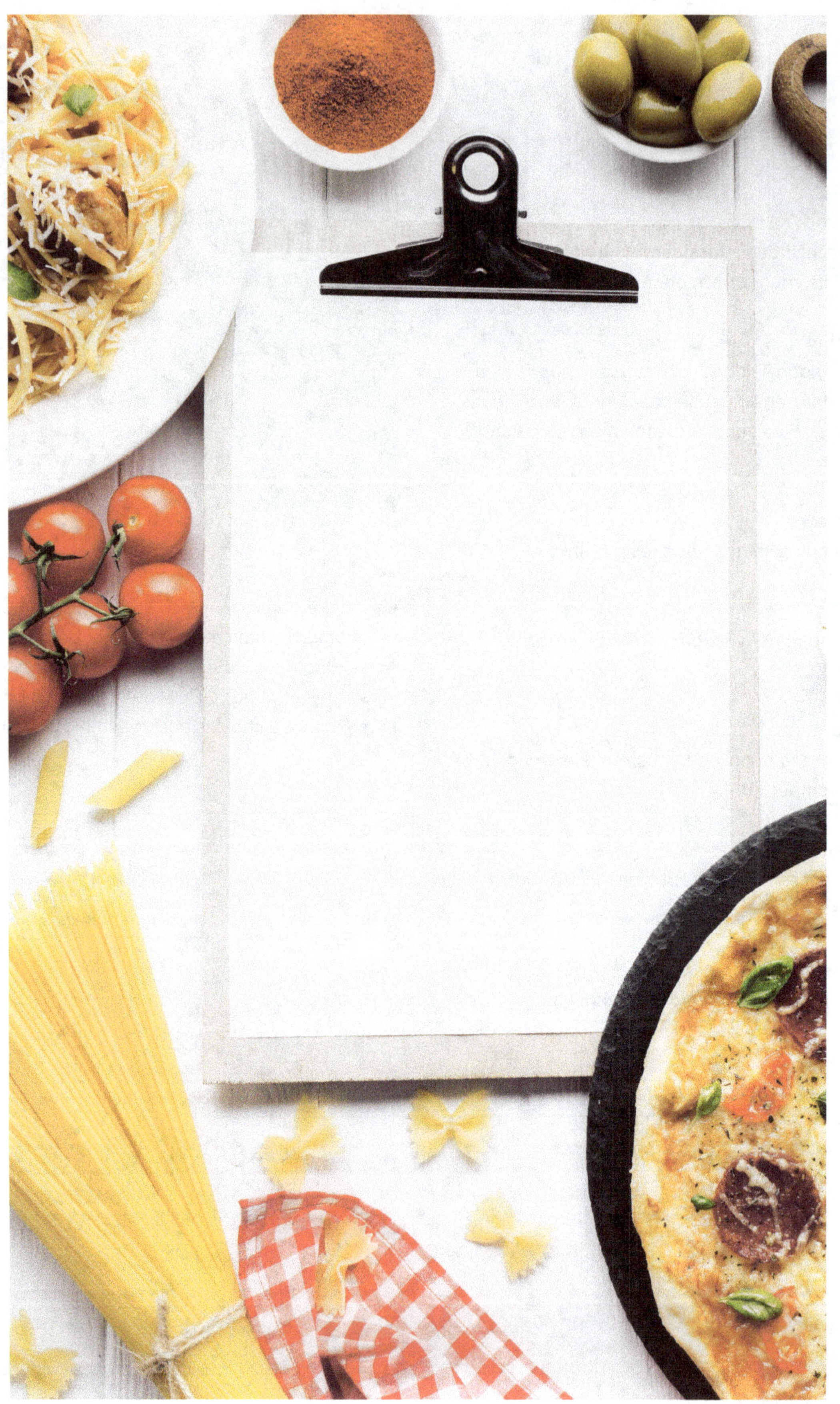

CHAPTER 1: CREATING YOUR PERSONAL SAFE FOOD LIST

Building Security Through Predictability

For many neurodivergent people, predictability is one of the most important parts of eating. When you know exactly how a food will taste, feel, and look every time, it can take away a lot of stress. Having a list of reliable, comfortable foods means you can always find something to eat without worry or pressure. This is your "safe food list," and it can be one of the most useful tools in your kitchen.

Emotional Validation

You might have heard criticism about eating the same foods repeatedly, but there is nothing wrong with finding comfort in predictability. Many neurotypical people have their own food routines, they just are not questioned about them. Whether your safe food list has twenty items or only three, it serves a real purpose. Feeling secure in your food choices is not a weakness. It is a form of self-care.

Understanding What Makes a Food "Safe"

A safe food is one you can eat without anxiety or unpleasant surprises. You know its texture, taste, smell, and appearance will be the same every time. It may be a specific brand, a certain cooking method, or even a particular plate or cup you always use. Safe foods are not "bad" foods or something to outgrow, they are essential tools for regulation and nourishment.
Safe foods often work because they do not overload your sensory system. When you know exactly how something will feel in your mouth, smell, and taste, your brain can focus on enjoying the meal instead of processing unexpected sensations.

Safe Food Categories and Common Patterns

Safe foods usually follow patterns. You might notice you prefer:

Specific textures: smooth, crunchy, chewy, or soft

Mild flavors: lightly salted, buttery, plain

Predictable shapes and colors: certain pasta shapes, crustless bread, peeled fruit

Familiar cooking methods: boiled, baked, or pan-fried in the same way each time

Trusted brands: because they deliver the exact flavor you expect

Recognizing these patterns can help you find new foods that are more likely to be accepted.

Building Your Personal Safe Food Inventory

Write down every safe food you can think of, no matter how few there are. Having only three to five safe foods is completely valid. Be specific. Instead of "bread," write "soft white sandwich bread, no seeds." Instead of "apples," write "peeled Honeycrisp apples, cut into thin slices." The more detail you include, the more helpful your list will be.

Organize your list by category:

Proteins (e.g., chicken tenders, mild cheese, peanut butter)

Carbs (e.g., white rice, plain pasta, soft rolls)

Fruits and Vegetables (if any are safe in certain forms)

Snacks (e.g., a specific brand of crackers, plain chips)

Drinks (e.g., chocolate milk, certain juices)

Working With Existing Preferences

Your safe foods are a foundation, not something to be "fixed." If you want to expand variety, you can do it slowly by making small changes that still keep the food mostly the same such as trying a slightly different pasta shape, a new breading on chicken tenders, or a brand of crackers that looks and tastes almost identical to your usual choice.

Safe foods can also change over time. A favorite food might fall off your list for no clear reason, and a new one might appear without warning. This is normal, and it is why keeping your list up to date is helpful.

Family Dynamics

If you are a parent, your child's safe foods might seem limited to you, but they serve an important purpose. Building trust around these foods first makes it easier to explore new ones later. Pressuring a child to abandon safe foods can backfire, but honoring those foods creates a sense of security that supports gentle growth over time.

Emergency Planning

It helps to have backup versions of safe foods on hand for days when your usual options are not available. Keep frozen, shelf-stable, or easy-to-find alternatives stocked. This can prevent stress during travel, illness, grocery shortages, or busy weeks.

Safe Food Discovery Worksheets

You can create a simple worksheet to track your safe foods and any new ones you try. Include:

- Name of the food
- Brand and preparation method
- Texture notes
- Temperature preference
- Whether it was a good match or not

This log can help you remember what works and avoid buying foods that did not feel right.

Expanding Within Safety Zones

When you are away from home: traveling, at someone else's house, or eating out, use your safe food list to look for "close matches." These are foods that share similar textures, colors, and flavors with your known safe foods. For example, if your safe food is soft white sandwich bread, a soft dinner roll might be a good match. If you like one brand of chicken nuggets, you might accept plain, lightly breaded chicken strips from a restaurant.

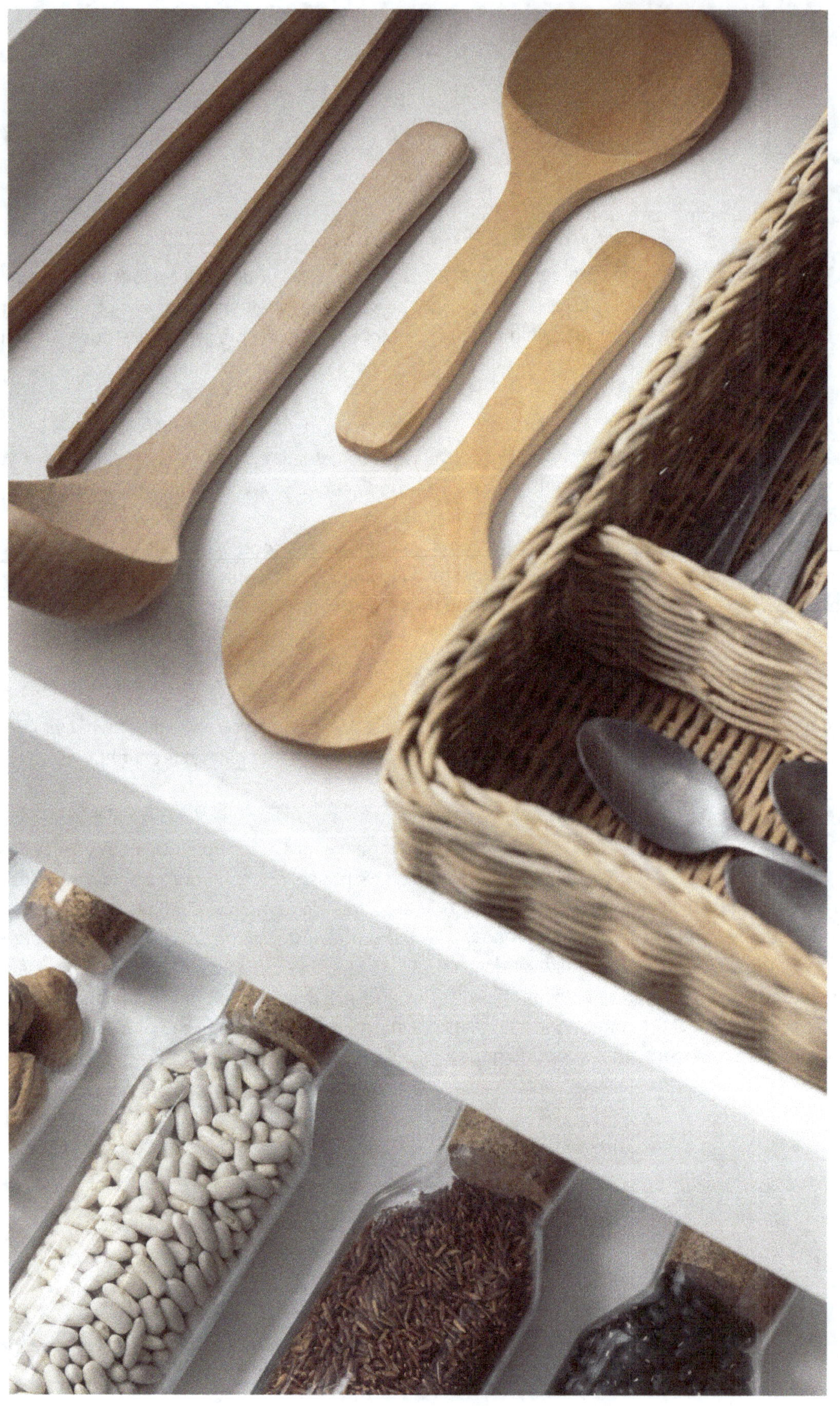

CHAPTER 2: KITCHEN SETUP FOR SUCCESS

The way your kitchen is arranged can have a big impact on how stressful or comfortable cooking feels. A space that feels overwhelming can drain your energy before you even start, while a calm, organized kitchen can make meals feel more manageable. The goal is not perfection, it's creating a setup that works for you, reduces stress, and helps you feel more in control.

Sensory-Friendly Kitchen Tools and Equipment

Some tools can help you avoid unpleasant textures, sounds, or smells while cooking:

- Disposable gloves or silicone-tipped tongs if you prefer not to touch raw meat, sticky dough, or other strong textures.
- Kitchen shears for cutting chicken, herbs, or other items without needing a cutting board.
- Silicone spatulas and utensils to reduce scraping noises.
- Electric can openers to avoid strain.
- Low-noise blenders or mixers if sound is a trigger.
- Nonstick pans to reduce scrubbing after cooking.

Organization Systems That Actually Work

Keeping your space organized saves time and reduces decision fatigue.

- Group items by category: breakfast foods together, snacks in one spot, baking supplies in one area.
- Store frequently used tools near where you use them most.
- Label shelves, drawers, and containers to help you quickly find and return items.
- Use clear containers or glass jars so you can see what you have at a glance.
- Take photos of your organized pantry or fridge to remember where things go.
- Use visual recipe cards or step-by-step photos for cooking instead of text-heavy instructions when possible.

Reducing Overwhelm in Food Prep Spaces

- Clear a small section of the counter as your "prep zone" before cooking.
- Only keep the tools and ingredients you need for the current recipe in that space.
- Cook in stages: prep ingredients, tidy up, then move to cooking.

Lighting Considerations

Good lighting makes it easier to see textures, colors, and doneness while reducing eye strain. If overhead lights feel too harsh, try softer under-cabinet lighting or a small lamp in your prep area.

Temperature Comfort

Cooking can heat up a kitchen quickly, which can lead to overwhelm. Use fans, open windows, or take short breaks to cool down. Adjust the space to stay at a temperature that feels comfortable to you.

Batch Prep Strategies

On high-energy days, make the most of your momentum:

- Wash and cut vegetables in advance.
- Cook a big pot of rice or pasta to use in multiple meals.
- Prepare proteins in batches so they are ready to reheat. Batch prepping saves time later and makes low-energy days easier.

Social Considerations

If you live with others, consider setting "quiet cooking times" where the kitchen is yours alone. This can reduce distractions, avoid sensory overload from extra voices or movement, and help you focus on the task.

Sound as a Kitchen Companion

Cooking can feel overwhelming when there are too many competing sounds or distractions in the background. One way to ease this is by bringing in a steady, predictable audio stream, whether that's music, a podcast, or an audiobook. For many neurodivergent individuals, the rhythm of familiar songs or the continuous flow of spoken words can anchor attention and make the task at hand less daunting. Research shows that spoken audio can help prevent the mind from wandering, especially during repetitive or less demanding kitchen tasks like chopping, stirring, or waiting for food to cook. In practice, this means the right soundtrack can reduce sensory stress, create a sense of focus, and even make food prep more enjoyable. Think of it as building an environment that propels you forward, one small step at a time.

Clean-As-You-Go Strategies for Executive Function

- Keep a bowl of warm, soapy water in the sink to drop used utensils in.
- Rinse and reuse tools for similar tasks during cooking.
- Wipe counters while food simmers or bakes.
- If cleaning mid-recipe is too distracting, set a short timer for cleanup after the meal.

Backup Plans for Bad Brain Days

Some days you may not be able to cook from scratch. Keep a list of low-effort meals you can make quickly, such as:

- Frozen safe meals.
- Pre-cooked proteins like grilled chicken breast strips.
- Microwaveable soups or pasta.
- Snack plates with protein, carbs, and fruit.
- Canned tuna or salmon with crackers or bread.
- Hard-boiled eggs (store-bought peeled or made ahead).

- Cheese and whole grain crackers with apple slices.
- Yogurt with fruit and granola.
- Instant oatmeal with milk and a spoonful of nut butter.
- Frozen vegetable stir-fry mix with pre-cooked protein, heated together.

Also keep pre-made safe foods from the grocery store on hand for times when energy is low. If possible, arrange for grocery delivery so you can restock without leaving home. You might also have a trusted friend or family member who can help with quick grocery runs in an emergency.

Emergency Food Storage and Rotation

Maintain an "emergency stash" of shelf-stable or frozen safe foods and rotate them regularly so they stay fresh:

- Shelf-stable pasta, crackers, or bread alternatives.
- Canned fruit in juice.
- Shelf-stable milk or milk alternatives.
- Frozen bread, muffins, or waffles.
- Frozen safe vegetables like peas or corn.

Success Tips: Troubleshooting Common Sensory Issues

- If touching raw meat is uncomfortable, use disposable gloves, a fork, or kitchen shears to handle and cut it without direct contact. You can also prep raw meat on parchment paper or in a shallow dish to reduce cleanup and avoid cross-contamination.
- If strong smells bother you, use the vent, open a window, or cook outdoors when possible.
- If loud kitchen noises are overwhelming, wear noise-reducing headphones or listen to calming background sounds.
- Use one-pot or one-pan recipes to limit multitasking and cleanup.
- Always use a timer to avoid overcooking when distracted.
- Keep a small trash bowl or compost container on the counter so you do not have to walk to the trash repeatedly while prepping.
- Set up ingredients before starting so you can cook without searching mid-recipe.
- Keep oven mitts, towels, and hot pads within arm's reach of your stove or oven to reduce rushed movements.
- If bright lights are uncomfortable, use softer lighting but keep enough illumination to see food safely.

- If you feel sensory overload building, turn off the stove or oven before leaving the kitchen, then take a short break to reset in a quieter space. This way you can regroup without worrying about leaving something unattended.
- Use pre-chopped or frozen vegetables and pre-cooked proteins to cut down on handling and prep time.
- If multitasking is difficult, focus on cooking one recipe at a time instead of juggling multiple dishes.

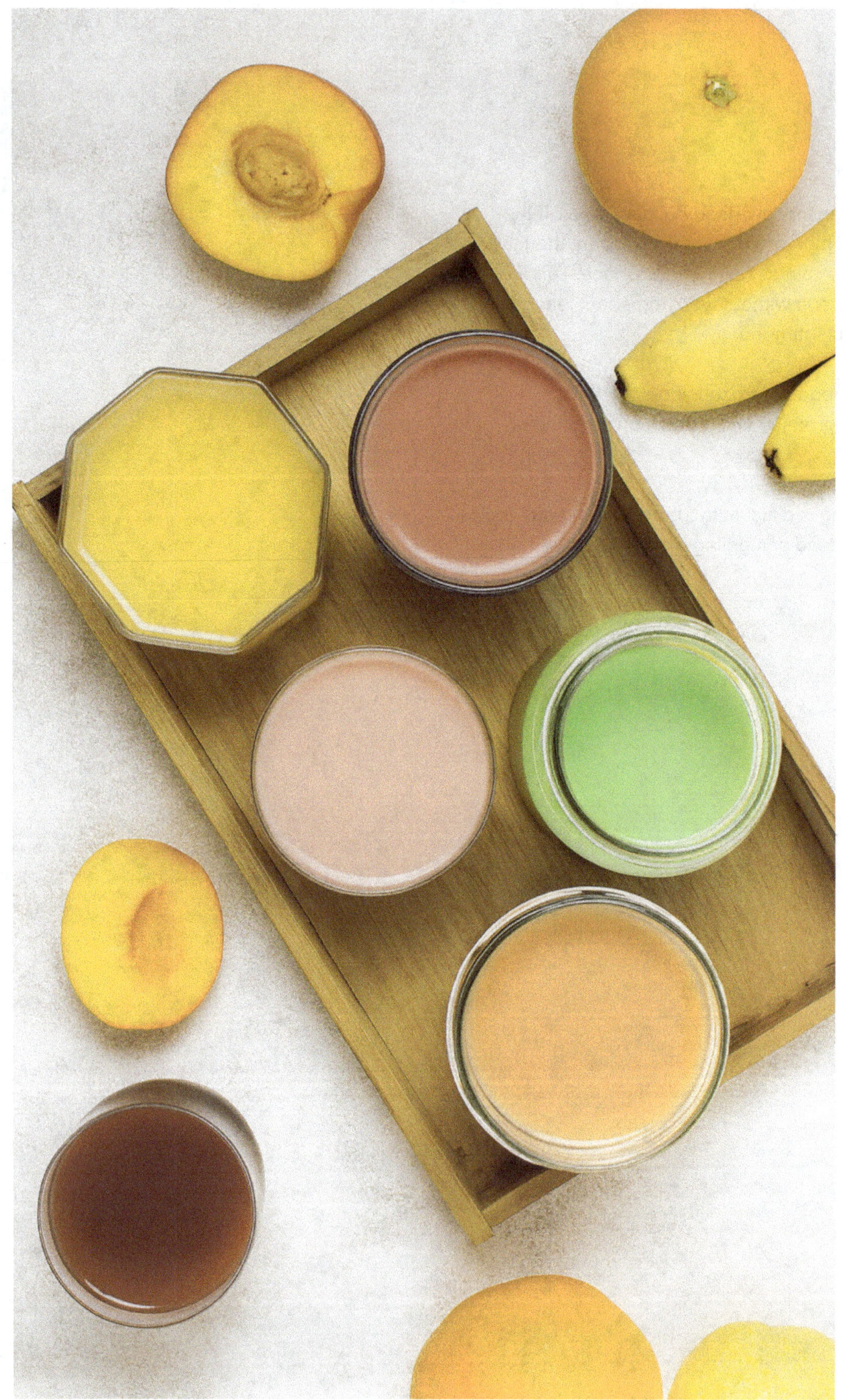

CHAPTER 3: SMOOTH SMOOTHIES AND JUICES

Smoothies can be a game-changer if fruits and vegetables are a sensory challenge for you. The right smoothie blends everything into a completely smooth, uniform texture, removing the lumps, pulp, or fibrous bits that can make certain foods hard to eat. These recipes are designed to be texture-free, so you can enjoy the flavors and nutrition without surprises in your mouth. They are also a gentle way to increase your intake of vitamins, minerals, protein, and fiber, even if eating these foods in their whole form doesn't work for you. Pre-slicing bananas, peaches, or other fruits before freezing makes them easier to blend and speeds up prep time. You can also buy pre-cut frozen fruits from the grocery store to skip peeling, chopping, and mess altogether. Having ready-to-use frozen produce on hand means you can make a nourishing smoothie in just minutes, without worrying about food going bad in the fridge.

Every recipe in this chapter has been tested to blend into a silky, clump-free drink that's easy to sip and easy to digest. There are no seeds, gritty powders, or stringy greens to deal with. You'll find classic flavors, comforting combinations, and hidden-veggie blends that mask stronger tastes, making it simple to get a balance of nutrients without forcing yourself to chew through textures you find uncomfortable. Whether you're starting your day, needing a quick snack, or looking for a soothing option on a low-energy afternoon, these smoothies can be prepared in minutes and enjoyed anywhere.

PERFECT VANILLA SMOOTHIE

Spoon Rating: 🍴🍴
Makes: 1 servings
Texture: Completely smooth
Temperature: Cold
Prep Time: 5 minutes
Calories per serving: ~250–350
Sensory Notes: Creamy, mild vanilla flavor with no seeds, lumps, or unexpected textures

This smoothie is simple, comforting, and perfect for days when you want something cold, creamy, and familiar. It's easiest to peel and slice the bananas before freezing so they blend more evenly. You can add vanilla protein powder for extra nutrition. If the tartness of yogurt is an issue, the banana and honey will soften those flavors. If you don't have frozen bananas, you can swap for a room temperature banana and extra ice. The uniform texture makes it a sensory-friendly option for anyone who avoids pulp, seeds, or lumps.

1 cup cold milk of choice (dairy or non-dairy)

1 frozen banana, peeled and sliced (or room temperature banana + ½ cup ice)

½ cup plain Greek or vanilla yogurt (dairy or non-dairy)

½ teaspoon pure vanilla extract

1 tablespoon honey or maple syrup (optional, for sweetness)

½ cup ice cubes (optional, for extra chill)

1. Pour the cold milk into the blender first so the blades run smoothly.
2. Add the sliced frozen banana, yogurt, honey or maple syrup (if using), and vanilla extract.
3. Add ice cubes if you want a thicker, frostier smoothie.
4. Blend on high for 45-60 seconds, scraping down the sides of the blender if needed to make sure there are no lumps.
5. Pour into a glass and enjoy immediately, or refrigerate for up to 12 hours.

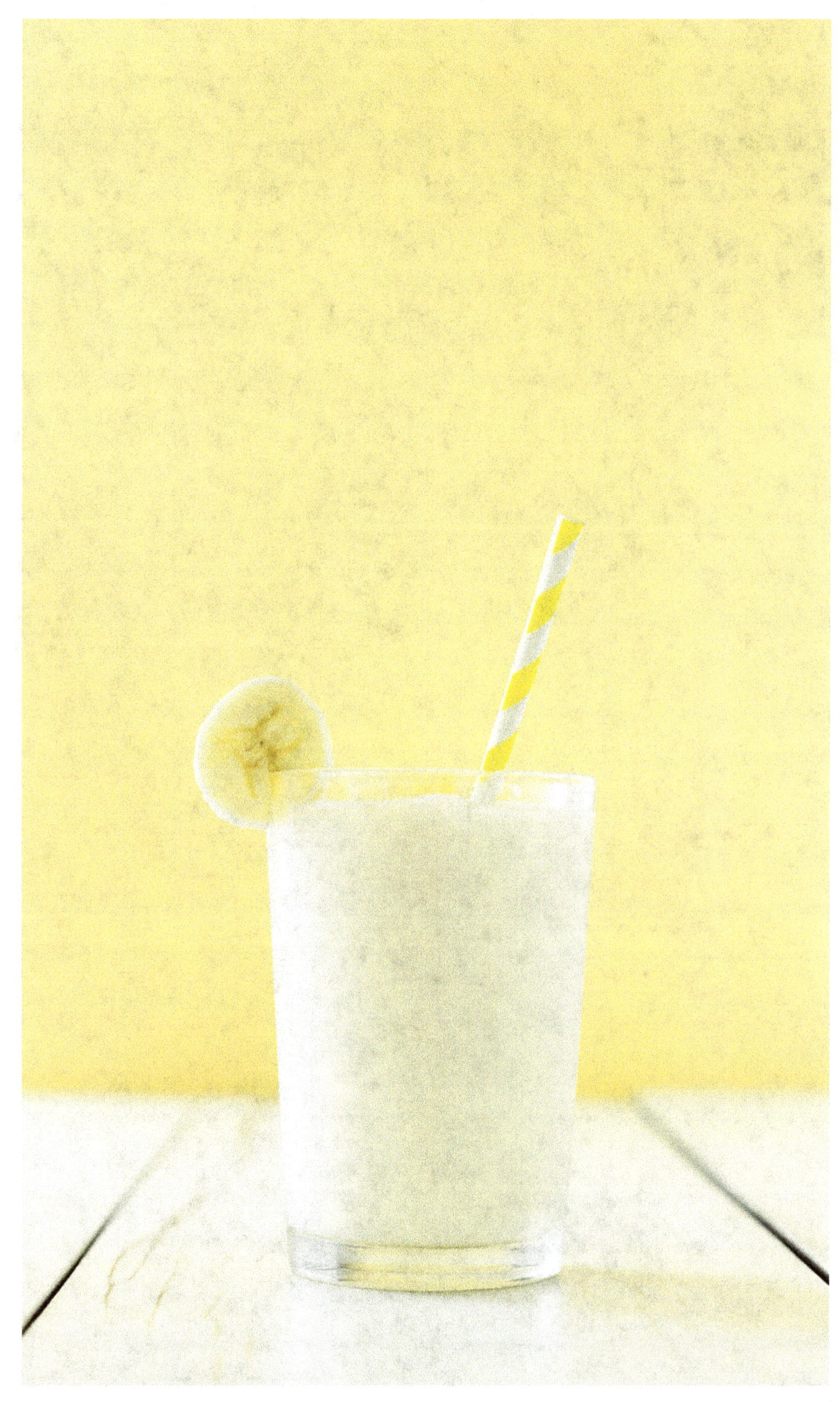

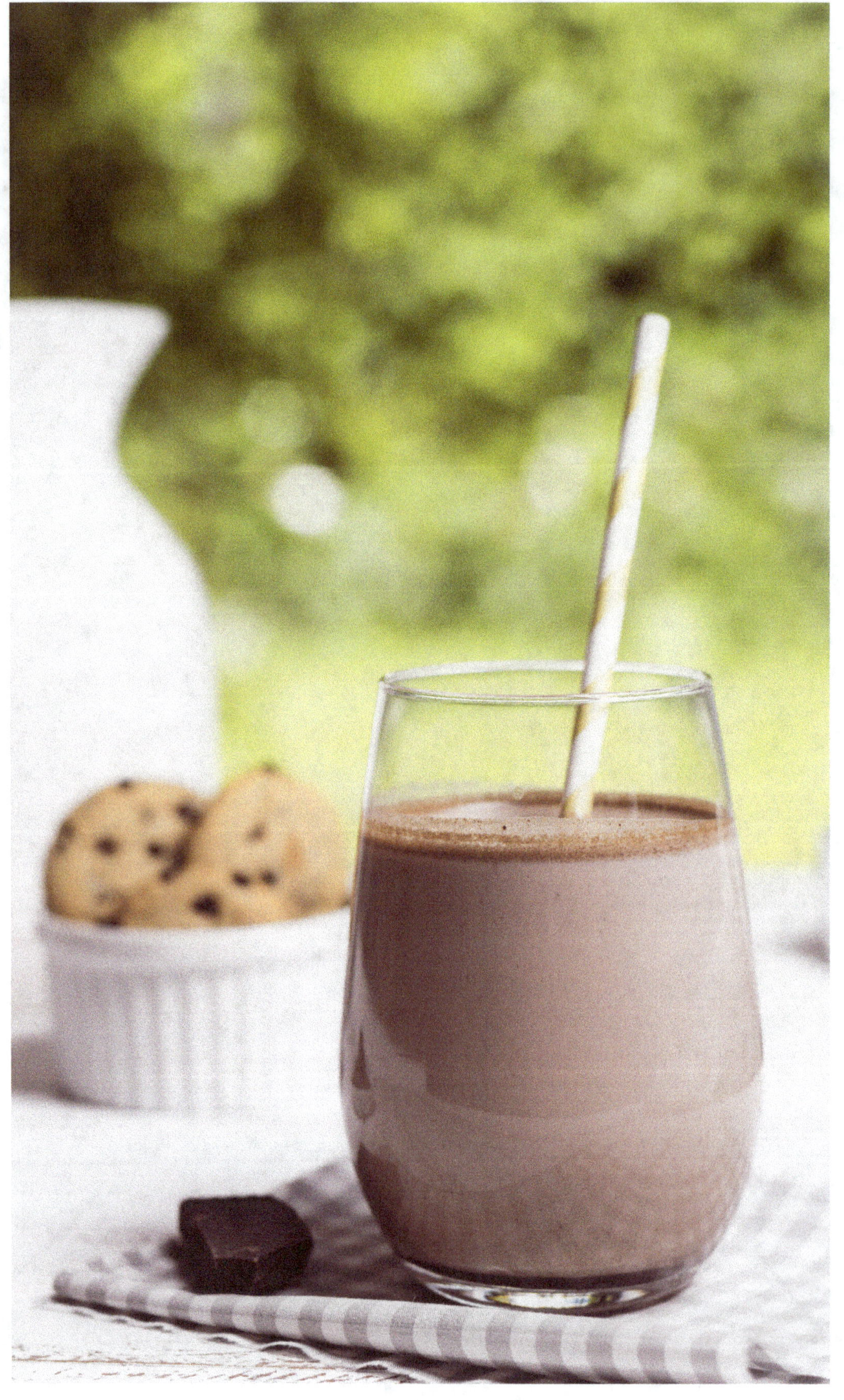

CHOCOLATE PEANUT BUTTER POWER SMOOTHIE

Spoon Rating: 🍴
Makes: 1 servings
Texture: Completely smooth
Temperature: Cold
Prep Time: 5 minutes
Calories per serving: ~350–450
Sensory Notes: Creamy, rich chocolate and peanut butter flavor with no chunks or grit

This smoothie tastes like dessert but is packed with protein and healthy fats to keep you full. Pre-slicing bananas before freezing makes blending easier and keeps the texture perfectly smooth. If you want extra nutrition, you can add a scoop of chocolate protein powder in place of the unsweetened cocoa powder. If frozen bananas aren't available, use a ripe room-temperature banana and add extra ice for chill. The rich, creamy texture makes this a great choice for anyone avoiding gritty or chunky drinks.

1 cup cold milk of choice (dairy or non-dairy)

1 frozen banana, peeled and sliced (or room temperature banana + ½ cup ice)

2 tablespoons peanut butter (creamy, not chunky)

1 tablespoon unsweetened cocoa powder

1 tablespoon honey or maple syrup (optional, for sweetness)

½ cup plain Greek or vanilla yogurt (dairy or non-dairy)

½ cup ice cubes (optional, for extra chill)

1. Pour the cold milk into the blender first.
2. Add the sliced frozen banana, peanut butter, cocoa powder, honey or maple syrup (if using), and yogurt.
3. Add ice cubes if you prefer a thicker, frostier smoothie.
4. Blend on high for 45-60 seconds, scraping down the sides if needed to ensure a completely smooth texture.
5. Pour into a glass and enjoy immediately, or refrigerate for up to 12 hours.

PEACH BANANA CLASSIC SMOOTHIE

Spoon Rating: ⍿⍿
Makes: 1 servings
Texture: Completely smooth
Temperature: Cold
Prep Time: 5 minutes
Calories per serving: ~250–350
Sensory Notes: Mild, sweet, fruity, with no pulp or chunks

This smoothie is light, sweet, and simple, perfect for when you want something fruity without any tang or bitterness. Precutting and freezing the peaches and banana makes blending fast and easy, and also helps create a naturally chilled, creamy texture. You can use store-bought frozen fruit to save time and reduce prep work. If fresh peaches are in season, slice and freeze them ahead for the best flavor.

1 cup frozen peach slices

1 medium frozen banana, sliced

1 cup cold milk of choice (dairy or non-dairy)

1 tablespoon honey or maple syrup (optional, adjust to taste)

½ teaspoon pure vanilla extract

1. Add the frozen peach slices, frozen banana slices, cold milk, honey or maple syrup (if using), and vanilla to a blender.
2. Blend on high until completely smooth, pausing to scrape down the sides of the blender if needed.
3. Taste and adjust sweetness, blending again briefly if you add more.
4. Pour into a glass and serve immediately.

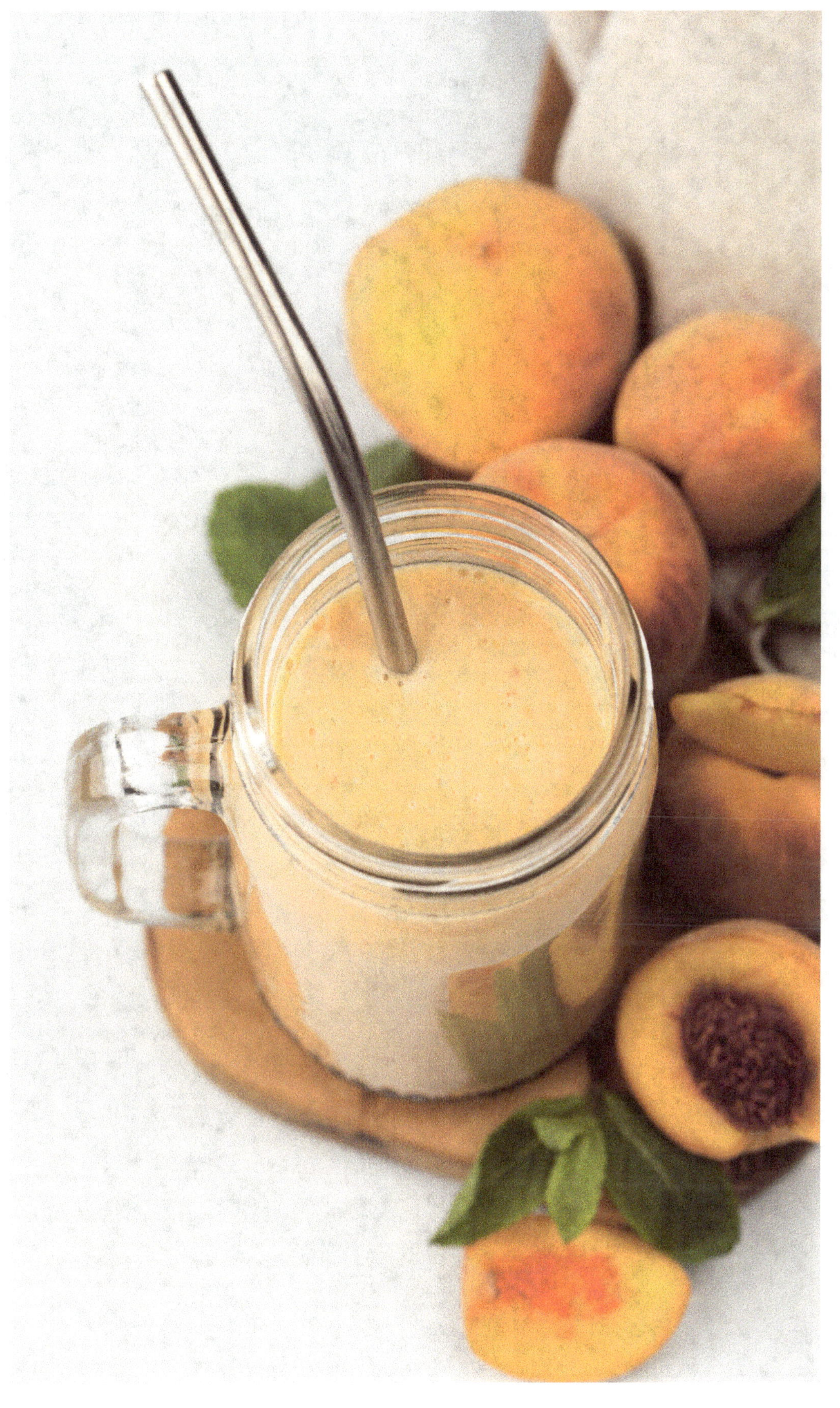

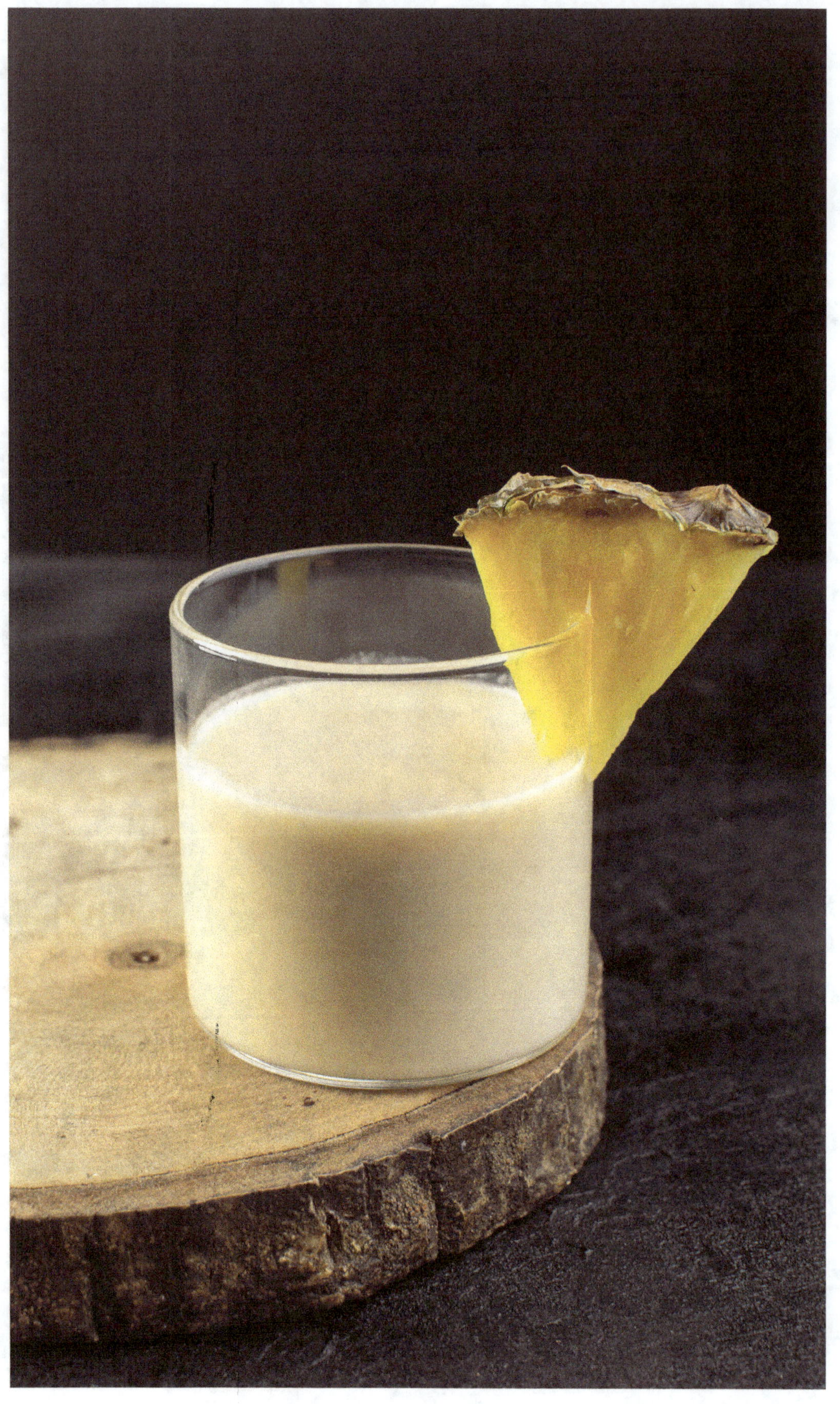

ANTI-ANXIETY PINEAPPLE SMOOTHIE WITH CHAMOMILE TEA

Spoon Rating: 🍴
Makes: 1 servings
Texture: Smooth and creamy
Temperature: Cold
Prep Time: 5 minutes (plus cooling time for tea)
Calories per serving: ~250–300
Sensory Notes: Sweet pineapple with calming floral undertones, silky and refreshing

This smoothie combines the calming effects of chamomile tea with the bright, tropical sweetness of pineapple. It's a soothing option for days when you feel overstimulated or anxious, offering a balance of gentle flavors and steadying nutrition.

1 cup strong brewed chamomile tea, cooled

1 ½ cups frozen pineapple chunks

1 ripe banana (fresh or frozen)

½ cup Greek yogurt (dairy or non-dairy)

1–2 teaspoons honey or maple syrup (optional, for extra sweetness)

½ cup cold milk of choice (dairy or non-dairy)

1. Brew chamomile tea according to the package directions and let it cool completely before using. (You can make extra and store in the fridge for easy smoothie prep.)
2. Add cooled chamomile tea, pineapple, banana, yogurt, honey (if using), and milk into a high-speed blender.
3. Blend on high until completely smooth. Scrape down the sides as needed to remove any clumps.
4. Taste and adjust sweetness if desired.
5. Serve immediately or chill in the fridge for up to 12 hours.

ROOM TEMPERATURE FRUIT JUICE

Spoon Rating: ⫶⫶⫶
Makes: 1 servings
Texture: Smooth, pulp-free option available
Temperature: Cold
Prep Time: 5 minutes
Calories per serving: ~150–180
Sensory Notes: Gentle sweetness, soft flavor, no cold shock

This juice is light, smooth, and easy to sip: perfect if cold drinks are uncomfortable or overwhelming. Using room-temperature fruit keeps the flavor gentle and avoids the sensory shock that comes with chilled or icy beverages. You can use fresh fruit straight from the counter or thaw frozen fruit in the fridge beforehand. Precutting fruit ahead of time makes it even easier to prepare.

1 cup chopped ripe peaches (fresh or thawed from frozen)

1 cup chopped ripe mango (fresh or thawed)

1 cup room-temperature water or coconut water

1 teaspoon honey or maple syrup (optional, adjust to taste)

1. Add peaches, mango, and water (or coconut water) to a blender.
2. Blend on high until completely smooth, scraping down the sides if needed.
3. Pour through a fine mesh strainer or cheesecloth into a glass for a pulp-free juice, or enjoy as-is for a thicker texture.

LIQUID MEAL REPLACEMENT SMOOTHIE

Spoon Rating: 🍴🍴
Makes: 1 servings
Texture: Smooth and creamy
Temperature: Cold
Prep Time: 5 minutes
Calories per serving: ~500–600
Sensory Notes: Mild banana-almond flavor, no grit, silky

This version is thick, silky, and satisfying, thanks to protein-rich Greek yogurt and healthy fats from almond butter. It's an easy way to get balanced nutrition when cooking isn't an option. Precut and freeze your bananas for quick prep and a naturally chilled drink, or use fresh bananas for a softer, less cold texture.

1 cup cold milk of choice (dairy or non-dairy)

½ cup plain Greek yogurt

1 medium banana (fresh or pre-cut frozen)

2 tablespoons almond butter (or peanut butter)

1 scoop chocolate or vanilla protein powder

1–2 teaspoons honey or maple syrup (optional)

1. Add all ingredients to a blender.
2. Blend on high until completely smooth, scraping down the sides if needed to remove any clumps.
3. Pour into a large glass and enjoy right away, or refrigerate for up to 12 hours.

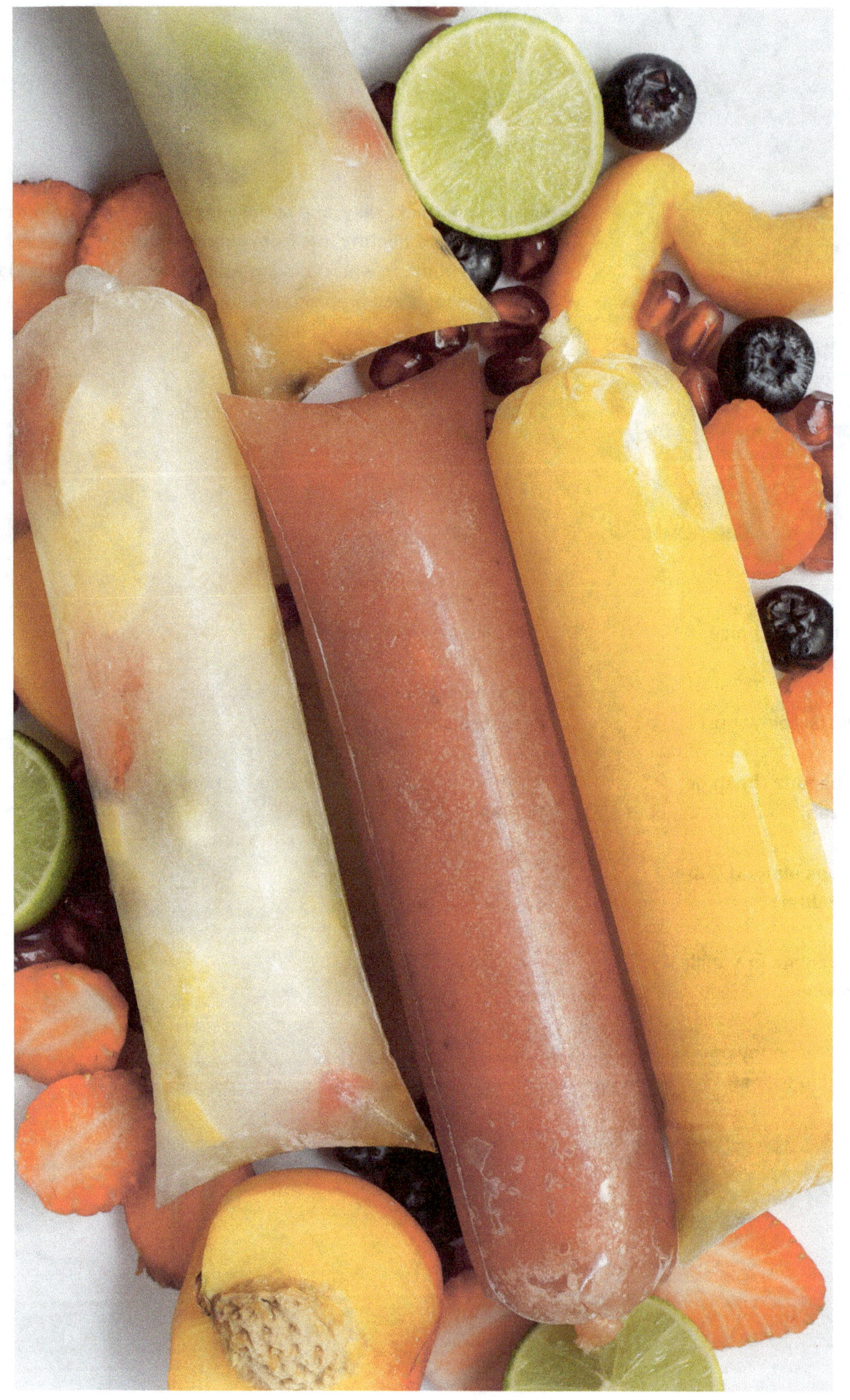

FREEZE-AHEAD FRUIT SMOOTHIE PACKS

Spoon Rating: 🍴🍴🍴
Makes: 1 servings
Texture: Smooth, minimal texture from berries
Temperature: Cold
Prep Time: 5 minutes (plus cooling time for tea)
Calories per serving: ~250–500
Sensory Notes: Bright and fruity

Freezer smoothie packs make it easy to have a nourishing drink ready anytime: just blend a large batch, portion into bags, jars, or ice pop sleeves, and freeze. Using pre-cut frozen fruit ensures a smooth, clump-free texture without unexpected seeds or fibers, making them ideal for sensory-sensitive eaters. They're customizable with your favorite flavors, last for weeks in the freezer, and give you instant, no-prep nutrition for busy mornings, post-workout recovery, or low-energy days.

Tropical Sunrise Smoothie

4 cups mango chunks
2 cups peaches
2 cups orange juice
1 cup coconut water

1. Add all ingredients to a high-speed blender.
2. Blend until completely smooth, pausing to scrape down the sides if needed.
3. Portion into freezer-safe containers and freeze.

Berry Citrus Burst

4 cups strawberries
2 cups blueberries
2 cups orange juice (cold)
1 cup pomegranate juice

1. Add all ingredients to a high-speed blender.
2. Blend until completely smooth, pausing to scrape down the sides if needed.
3. Portion into freezer-safe containers and freeze.

Watermelon Lime Cooler

4 cups watermelon chunks (seedless or remove seeds)
2 tablespoons fresh lime juice
2 cups cold apple juice (or coconut water for lighter flavor)

1. Add all ingredients to a high-speed blender.
2. Blend until completely smooth, pausing to scrape down the sides if needed.
3. Portion into freezer-safe containers and freeze.

GREEN JUICE THAT DOESN'T TASTE GREEN

Spoon Rating: 🥄🥄🥄
Makes: 1-2 servings
Texture: Silky and light
Temperature: Cold
Prep Time: 10 minutes
Calories per serving: ~150–180
Sensory Notes: Sweet and citrusy, no grassy aftertaste, refreshing finish

This juice is all about balance. Sweet fruits mask the strong flavors of leafy greens, so you get all the nutrition without the earthy taste. It's perfect if you want the benefits of greens but struggle with sensory overload from bitter or fibrous textures.

2 cups cold green grapes (seedless)

1 medium green apple, cored and chopped

1 cup cucumber, peeled and chopped

1 packed cup baby spinach (mild, soft leaves)

½ cup pineapple chunks (fresh or frozen, thawed)

Juice of ½ lemon or lime

1 cup cold water or coconut water

1. Wash and prepare all produce. If using frozen pineapple, let it thaw slightly.
2. Add grapes, apple, cucumber, spinach, pineapple, lemon juice, and water to a high-speed blender.
3. Blend until completely smooth. Pause and scrape down the sides if needed to eliminate pulp or small bits.
4. Strain through a fine mesh sieve if you prefer an ultra-smooth, pulp-free drink.
5. Pour into glasses and enjoy immediately, or store in sealed jars in the fridge for up to 24 hours.

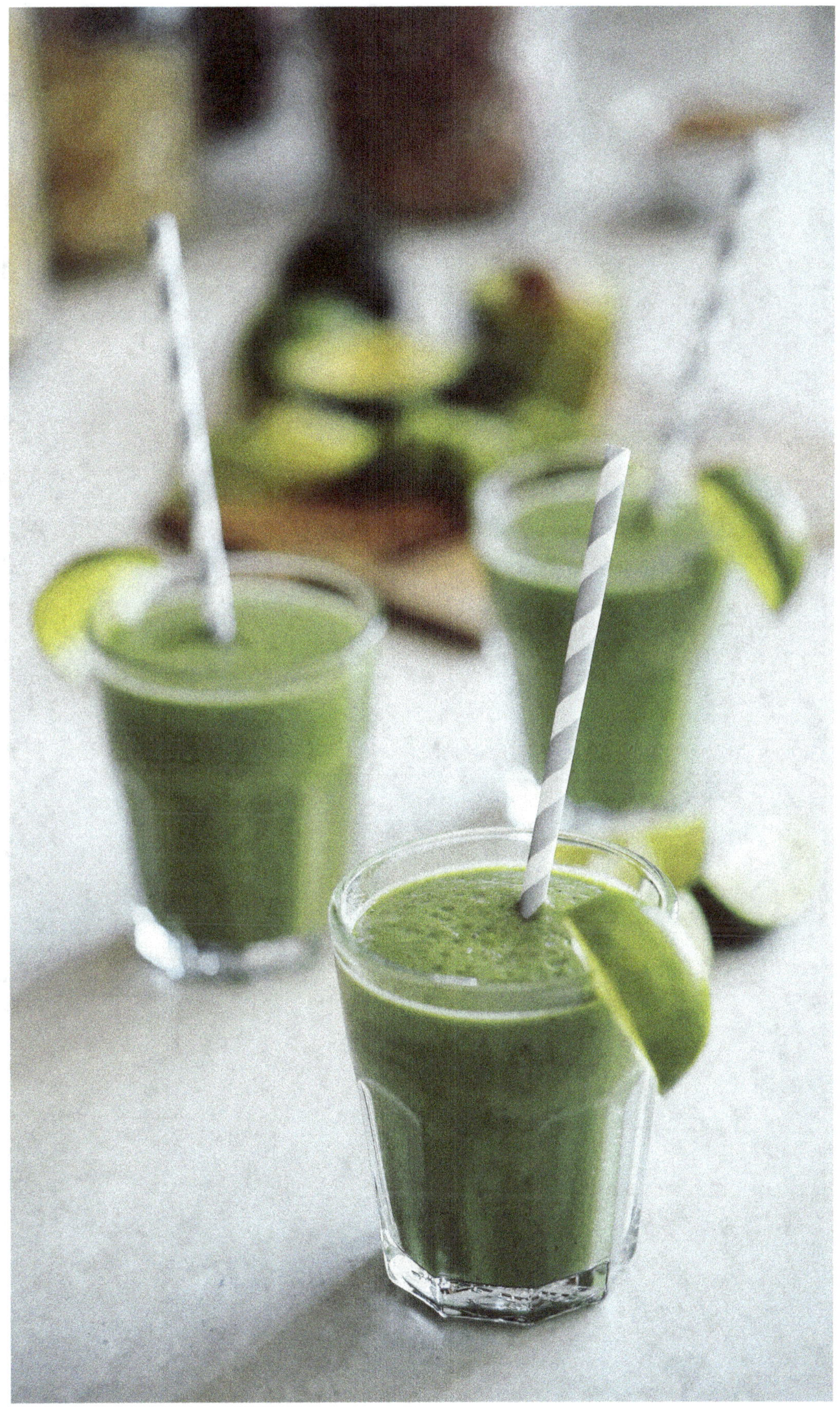

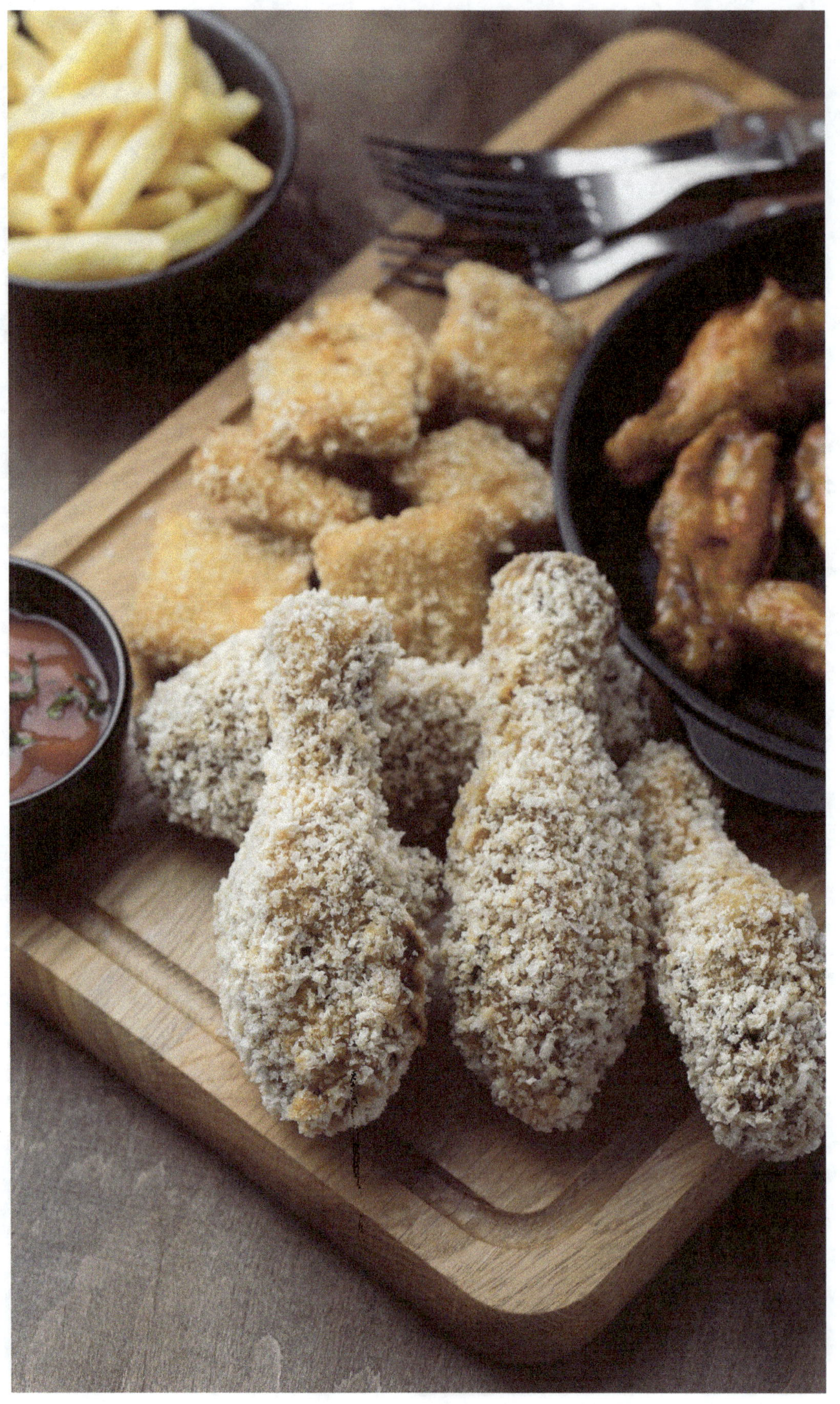

CHAPTER 4: IT'S ALL ABOUT THE CHICKEN

Chicken is one of the best proteins for neurodivergent eaters because it is both neutral in flavor and consistent in texture. Unlike foods that can surprise you with unexpected crunch, grit, or bitterness, chicken tends to taste mild and feel predictable bite after bite. It's also versatile: you can eat it plain, shred it into rice or pasta, or pair it with a gentle sauce. That reliability makes it easier to come back to again and again, especially if your food preferences shift or if you're struggling with safe options.

The challenge is that raw meat can be unpleasant to touch and hard to manage. If handling chicken is overwhelming, you don't have to force yourself. Use disposable gloves, tongs, or even kitchen scissors so you never need to touch it directly. Better yet, most raw meat can be bought already precut, or you can ask the butcher to cut it for you. This chapter will guide you through easy, low-stress ways to prepare and enjoy chicken, so you can get the nutrition without the sensory overload.

PERFECT BREADED CHICKEN TENDERS

Spoon Rating: ⍊⍊⍊⍊
Makes: 3–4 servings
Texture: Crispy outside, tender inside
Temperature: Hot
Prep Time: 20 minutes
Calories per serving: ~350–400
Sensory Notes: Mild flavor, crunchy coating, reliable bite

Chicken tenders are a comfort food classic, but they're also great for make-ahead prep. You can cook a big batch, freeze them, and then reheat whenever you need a quick, reliable meal. Using plain breadcrumbs and simple seasonings gives you a crispy outside with a tender, juicy inside that's easy to eat. If handling raw chicken feels like too much, use disposable gloves or tongs, or even ask the butcher to cut the chicken strips for you so prep feels less stressful.

1 lb chicken breast, sliced into strips (or buy precut chicken tenders)

1 cup plain breadcrumbs

½ cup all-purpose flour

2 eggs, beaten

1 teaspoon salt

½ teaspoon pepper (optional, mild flavor)

½ teaspoon garlic powder (optional, mild flavor)

½ teaspoon paprika (optional, mild flavor)

2–3 tablespoons neutral oil (for pan frying) or cooking spray (for baking)

1. If cutting your own chicken, slice breasts into even strips. If possible, buy precut tenders to save time and avoid handling.
2. Set up three bowls: one with flour, one with beaten eggs, and one with breadcrumbs mixed with salt (and optional seasonings, if using).
3. Coat each chicken strip in flour, then dip in egg, then coat fully in breadcrumbs. Place on a plate.
4. To pan fry: heat oil in a large skillet over medium heat. Cook tenders for 3–4 minutes per side until golden brown and fully cooked (internal temp 165°F).
5. To bake: preheat oven to 400°F (200°C). Place tenders on a parchment-lined sheet, spray lightly with cooking spray, and bake for 18–20 minutes, flipping halfway.
6. To air-fry: preheat to 375°F (190°C). Arrange tenders in single later and spray lightly with cooking spray. Cook for 10-12 minutes, flipping halfway, until golden brown and cooked through.
7. To freeze and reheat, let cooked tenders cool completely, then place in a freezer bag or airtight container. Reheat in the oven or airfryer at 375°F (190°C) for 10–15 minutes, or until hot and crisp.

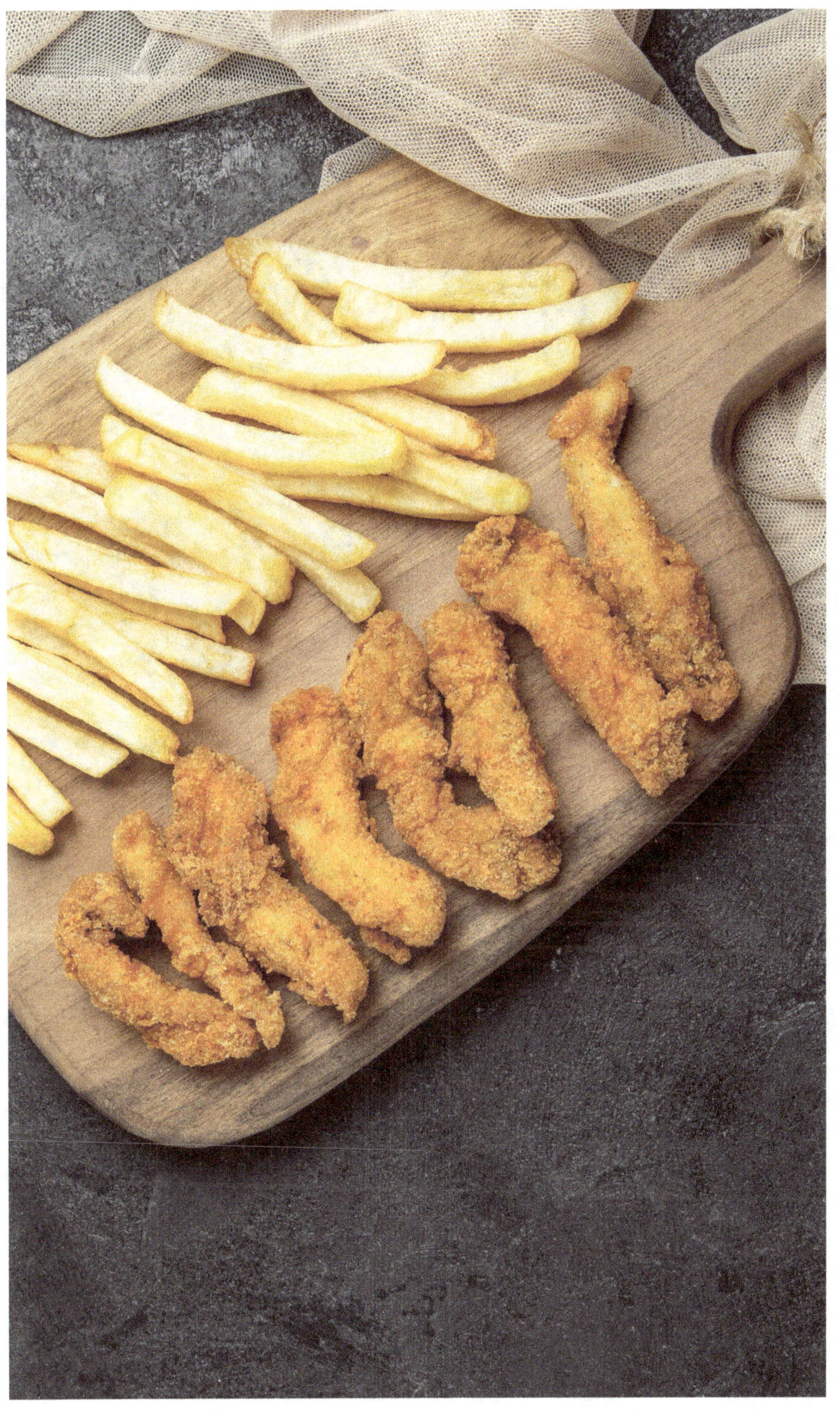

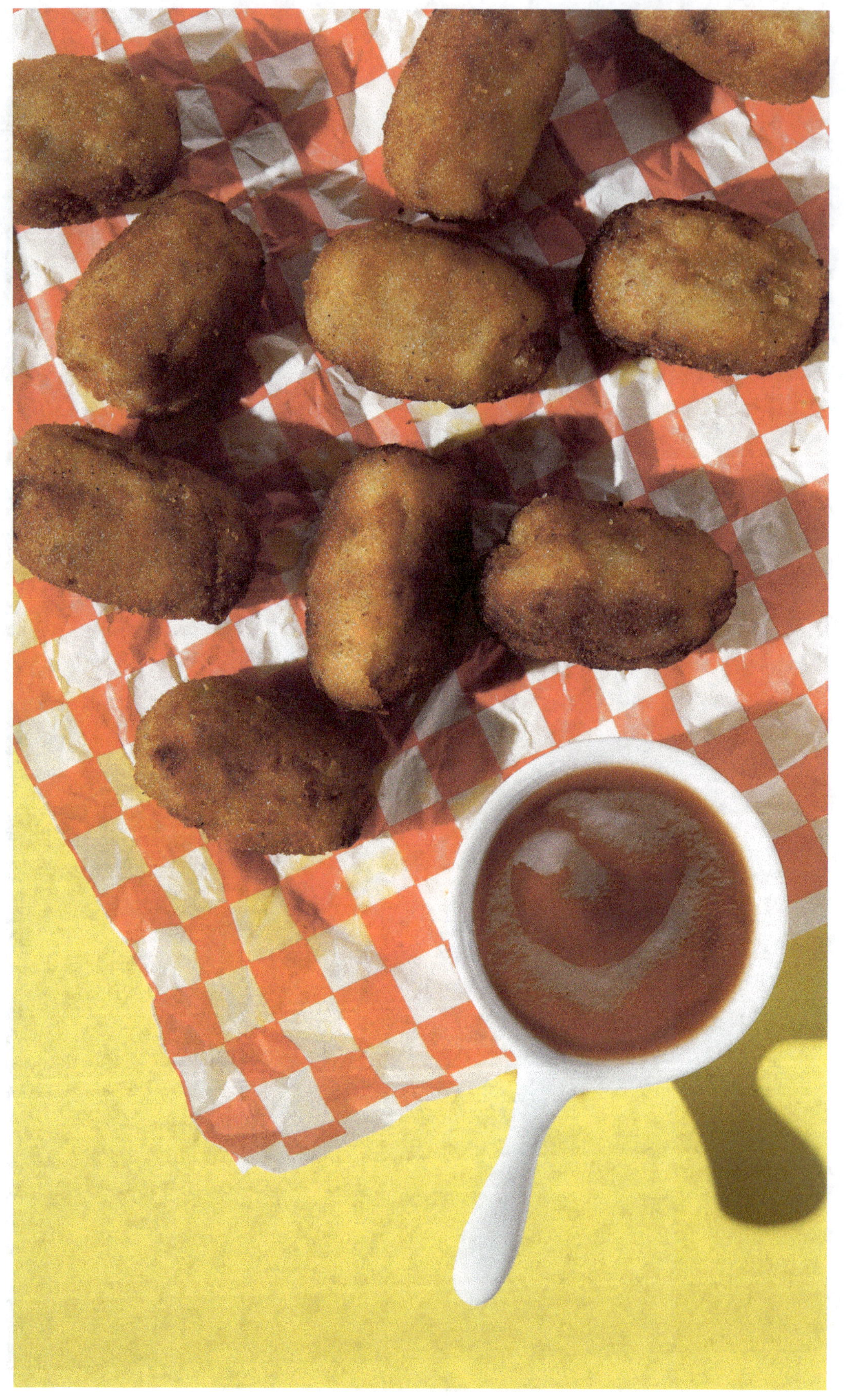

CRISPY BAKED CHICKEN NUGGETS

Spoon Rating: ⍿⍿⍿⍿
Makes: 3–4 servings
Texture: Crunchy outside, tender inside
Temperature: Hot
Prep Time: 20 minutes
Calories per serving: ~300–350
Sensory Notes: Mild flavor, small manageable pieces, consistent texture

Chicken nuggets are a comfort food that feel safe, familiar, and easy to eat. Making them at home gives you control over flavor and texture, while still keeping prep simple. You can even double or triple the recipe and freeze extras for quick reheating later. If handling raw chicken feels overwhelming, ask the butcher to precut the pieces for you, or use disposable gloves and tongs. These nuggets use plain breadcrumbs with optional mild seasonings, giving you a crunchy outside and tender inside that works for selective eaters while still being satisfying for everyone.

1 lb chicken breast, cut into bite-sized pieces (or buy precut from butcher)

1 cup plain breadcrumbs

½ cup all-purpose flour

2 eggs, beaten

1 teaspoon salt

½ teaspoon pepper (optional, mild flavor)

½ teaspoon garlic powder (optional, mild flavor)

½ teaspoon paprika (optional, mild flavor)

Cooking spray or 2 tablespoons neutral oil

1. Place flour in a large zip-top bag. Add chicken pieces, seal, and shake until evenly coated.
2. Transfer chicken pieces to the egg bowl, coating fully.
3. Dip each piece into breadcrumbs mixed with salt and seasonings, pressing gently so coating sticks. Place on a parchment-lined baking sheet or air fryer basket.
4. To bake: preheat oven to 400°F (200°C). Place nuggets on a parchment-lined sheet, spray lightly with cooking spray, and bake for 18–20 minutes, flipping halfway.
5. To air fry: Preheat air fryer to 375°F (190°C). Arrange nuggets in a single layer, spray lightly with cooking spray, and cook 10–12 minutes, shaking basket or flipping halfway, until golden and crisp.
6. To freeze and reheat, let cooked nuggets cool completely, then freeze in a single layer on a tray before transferring to a bag or airtight container. Reheat in oven or air fryer at 375°F (190°C) for 10–15 minutes until hot and crispy again.

PLAIN POACHED CHICKEN BREAST

Spoon Rating: 🍴🍴🍴
Makes: 2–3 servings
Texture: Soft, moist, consistent
Temperature: Hot (or chilled if storing)
Prep Time: 20 minutes
Calories per serving: ~200
Sensory Notes: Mild flavor, tender bite, reliable and versatile

Poached chicken is one of the easiest ways to cook chicken without dealing with breading, frying, or heavy seasoning. It's especially helpful for neurodivergent eaters because the texture is soft and consistent, and the flavor stays neutral. You can use it plain, chop it into small bites, or shred it for other recipes. If handling raw chicken feels stressful, wear disposable gloves, use tongs, or ask the butcher to cut the chicken for you so it's ready to drop straight into the pot. This recipe also works great for batch cooking: make a few breasts at once and store them in the fridge or freezer for quick meals later.

1–2 chicken breasts (about 1 lb, whole or precut by butcher)

4 cups water or mild chicken broth

1 teaspoon salt

Optional: 1 bay leaf, 2–3 slices of ginger, or a small piece of garlic or onion (for light flavor)

1. Place chicken breasts in a medium pot and cover with water or broth. Add salt and any optional aromatics.
2. Bring liquid just to a gentle simmer over medium heat. Do not boil (boiling can toughen the chicken).
3. Once simmering, reduce heat to low. Cover and cook 12–15 minutes, until chicken is opaque and internal temperature reaches 165°F (74°C).
4. Remove chicken from pot and let rest 5 minutes before slicing, dicing, or shredding.
5. To freeze and reheat, let chicken cool completely, then slice or shred. Store in airtight containers or freezer bags. Reheat gently in the microwave with a splash of broth or water to keep moist.

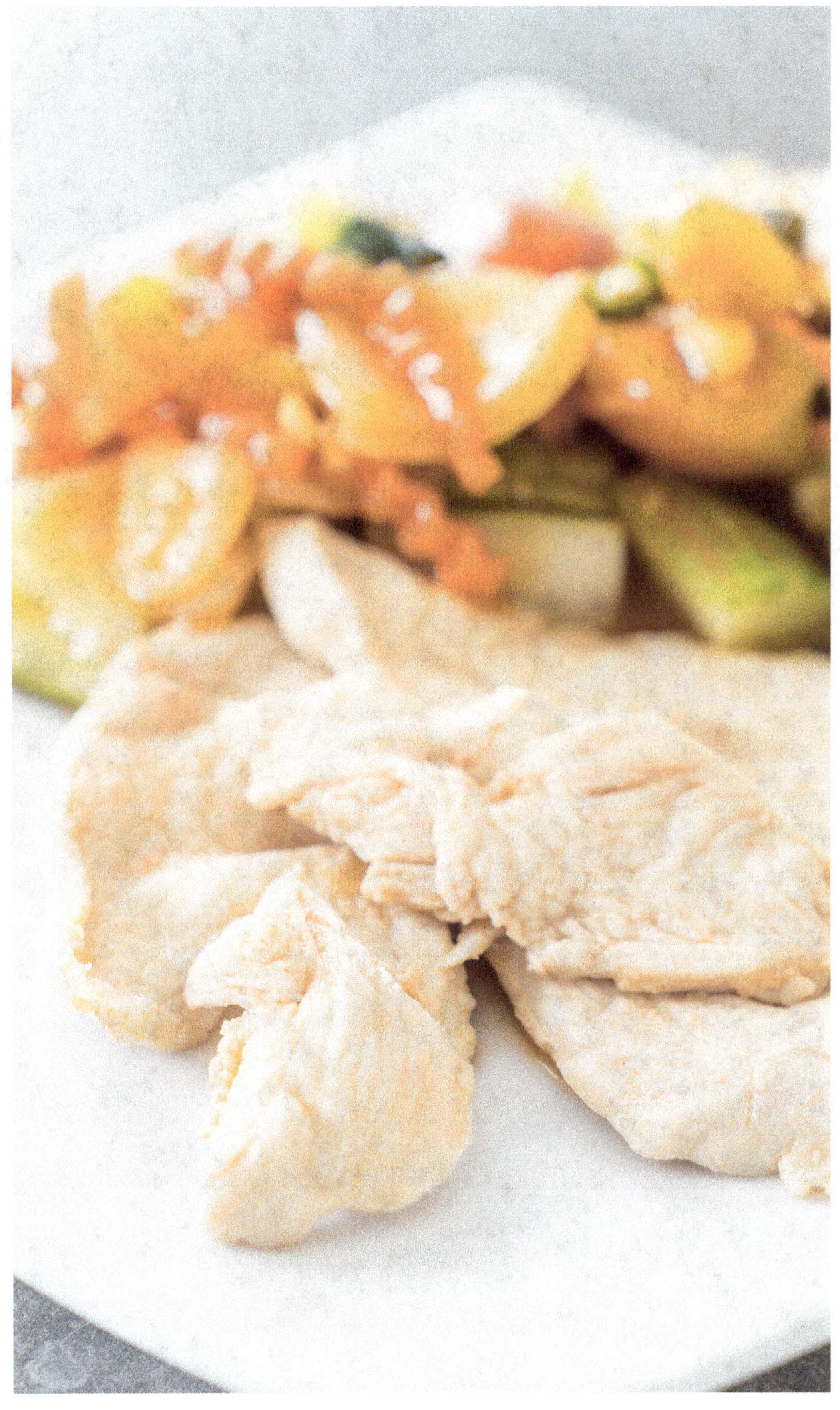

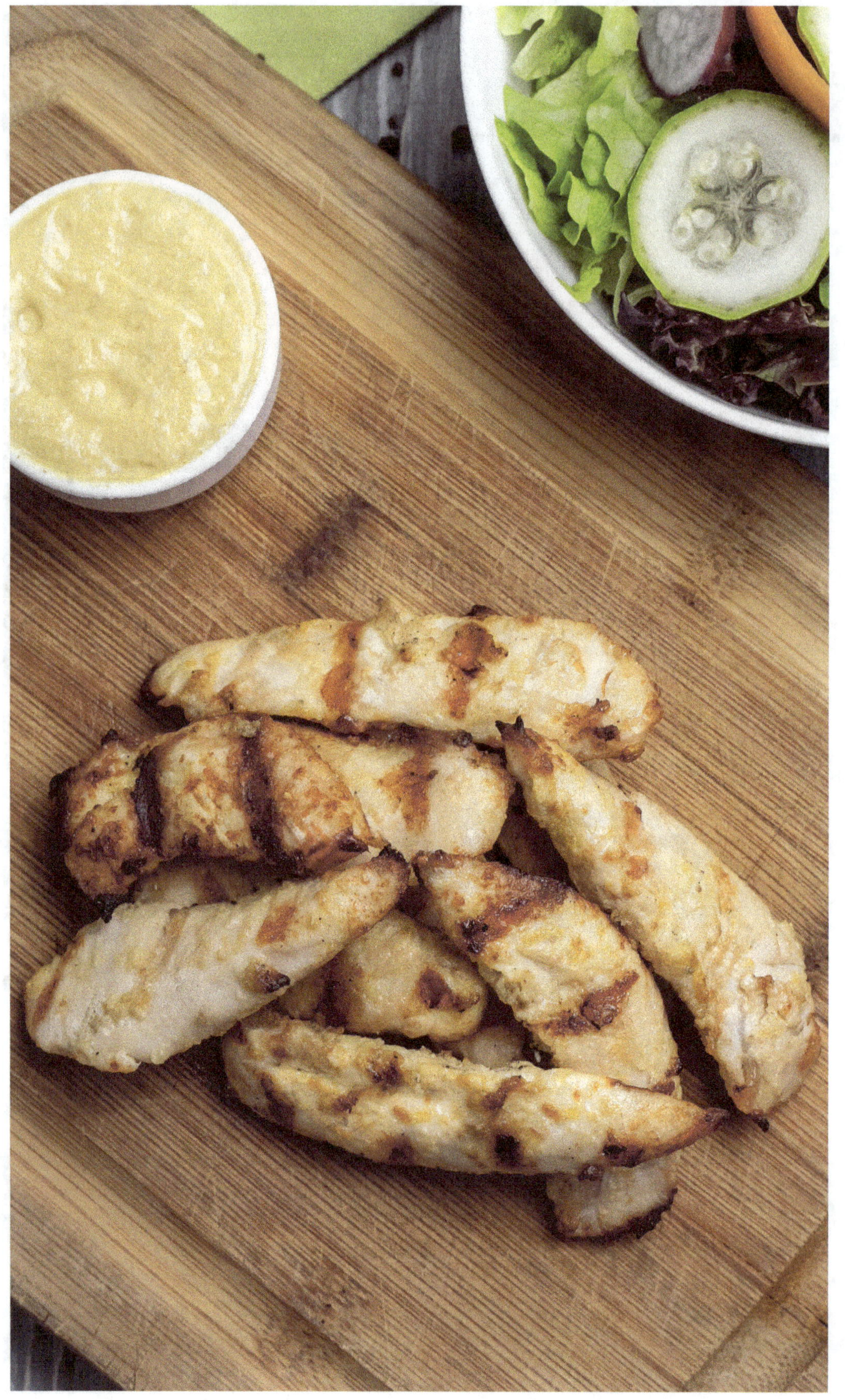

GRILLED CHICKEN STRIPS

Spoon Rating: 🍴🍴🍴
Makes: 3–4 servings
Texture: Juicy, slightly charred edges
Temperature: Hot
Prep Time: 20 minutes
Calories per serving: ~250–280
Sensory Notes: Mild flavor, smoky if outdoor-grilled, consistent bite

Grilled chicken strips are a simple, versatile option for quick meals. The flavor is mild but satisfying, and you can cook them either outdoors on a grill for smoky depth or indoors on a stovetop grill pan for convenience. They're easy to portion, reliable in texture, and work well on their own or as part of salads, wraps, or bowls. If handling raw chicken feels difficult, wear disposable gloves, use tongs, or ask the butcher to precut strips for you so they're ready to season and cook.

1 lb chicken breast, sliced into strips (or buy precut strips)

2 tablespoons olive oil or neutral oil

1 teaspoon salt

½ teaspoon pepper (optional, mild flavor)

½ teaspoon garlic powder (optional, mild flavor)

1. Place chicken strips in a bowl or zip-top bag and add oil, salt, and optional seasonings. Toss until evenly coated.
2. To grill indoors: heat a grill pan over medium-high heat. Lightly oil the surface, then cook strips 3–4 minutes per side until cooked through.
3. To grill outdoors: preheat grill to medium-high heat. Place chicken strips directly on the grates and cook 3–4 minutes per side until golden with grill marks and internal temp reaches 165°F (74°C).

PANKO BREADED CHICKEN DRUMSTICKS

Spoon Rating: ꟾꟾꟾꟾ
Makes: 3–4 servings
Texture: Extra crispy outside, juicy inside
Temperature: Hot
Prep Time: 15 minutes
Calories per serving: ~300–350
Sensory Notes: Crunchy coating, mild flavor, satisfying bite

Chicken drumsticks are a budget-friendly, hands-on favorite, and using panko breadcrumbs gives them an extra light and crispy coating. Panko is a Japanese-style breadcrumb that's larger and flakier than regular breadcrumbs, so it stays crunchier after baking. That makes it perfect for anyone who likes a crisp texture without heavy seasoning. If you prefer to avoid handling raw chicken, wear gloves, use tongs, or ask your butcher to prep the drumsticks for you so they're ready to coat and bake.

6 chicken drumsticks (skin on or off, your preference)

1 cup panko breadcrumbs

½ cup all-purpose flour

2 eggs, beaten

1 teaspoon salt

½ teaspoon pepper (optional, mild flavor)

½ teaspoon garlic powder (optional, mild flavor)

½ teaspoon paprika (optional, mild flavor)

Cooking spray or 2 tablespoons neutral oil

1. Pat drumsticks dry with a paper towel.
2. Place flour in a zip-top bag. Add drumsticks, seal, and shake until evenly coated.
3. Dip each drumstick into bowl with beaten egg, then in a separate bowl, roll in panko mixed with salt and optional seasonings. Press lightly so crumbs stick.
4. To bake: preheat oven to 400°F (200°C). Place drumsticks on a parchment-lined baking sheet, spray or drizzle with oil, and bake for 35–40 minutes, flipping halfway, until coating is golden and internal temp reaches 165°F (74°C).
5. To air-fry: preheat to 375°F (190°C). Arrange drumsticks in a single layer, spray with cooking spray, and cook 20–25 minutes, turning halfway, until crisp and cooked through.

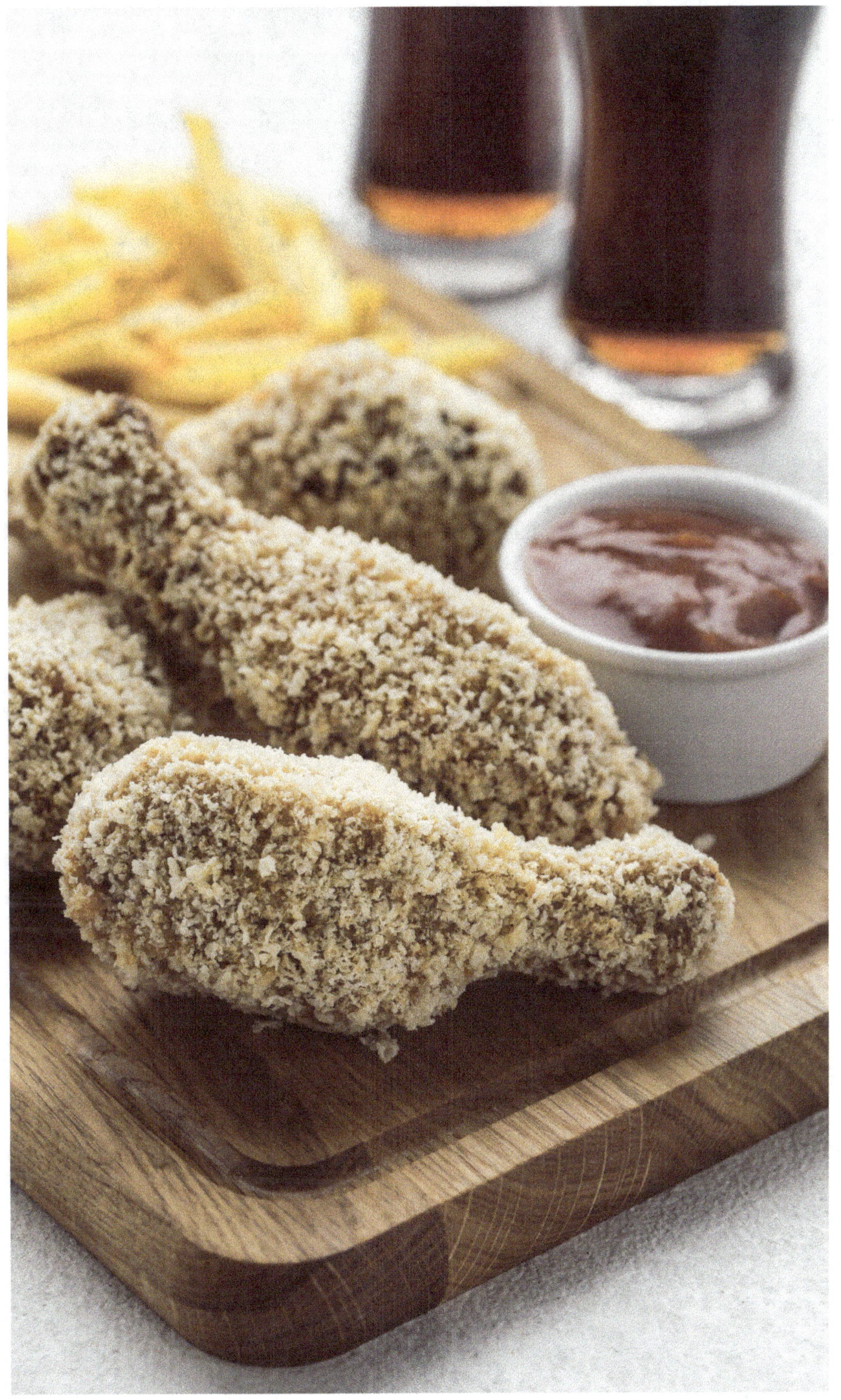

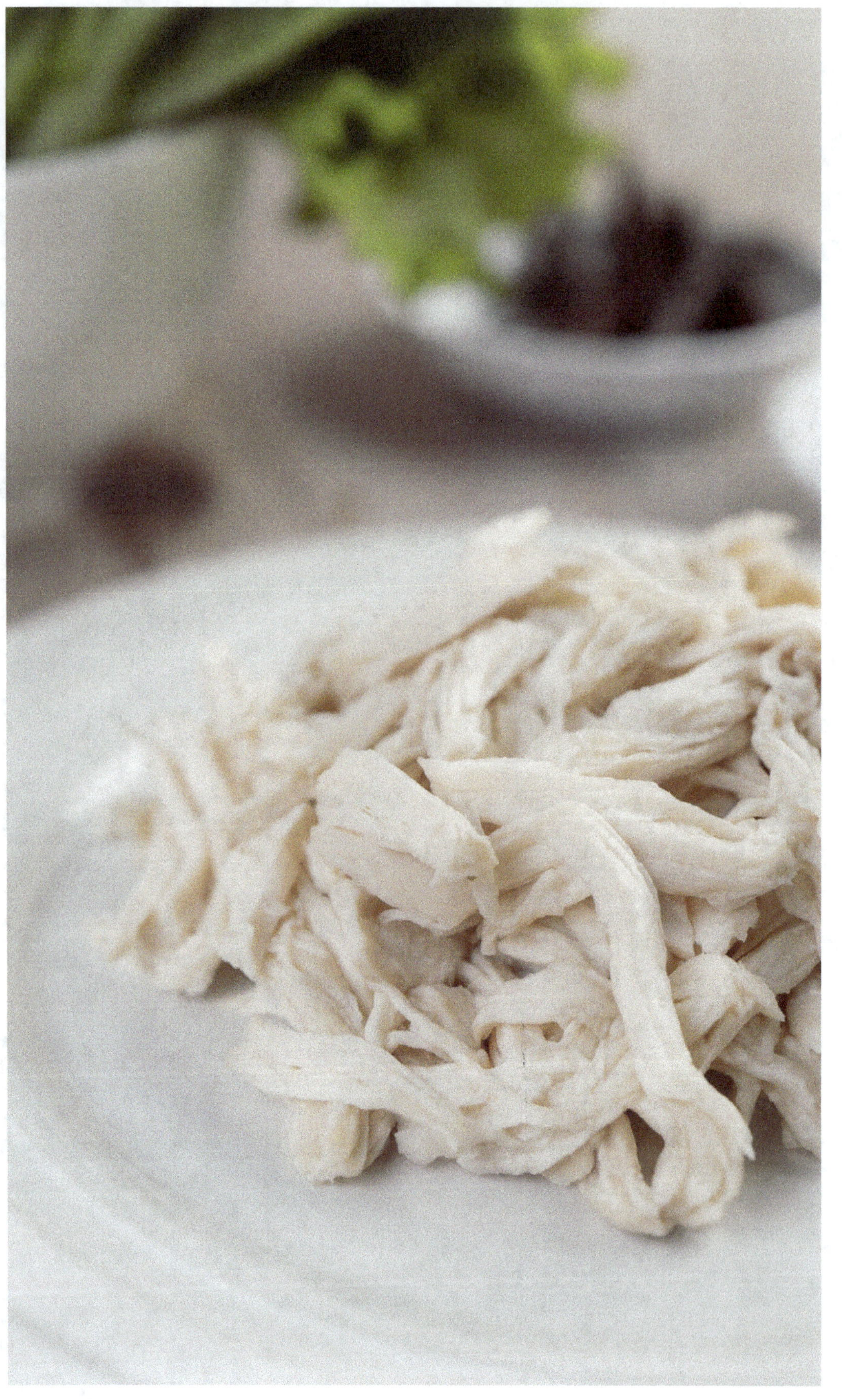

SLOW COOKER SHREDDED CHICKEN

Spoon Rating: 🍴🍴
Makes: 6–8 servings
Texture: Soft, stringy, moist
Temperature: Hot
Prep Time: 5 minutes
Calories per serving: ~200
Sensory Notes: Mild flavor, moist and tender, no strong seasoning

Shredded chicken is one of the easiest, most versatile ways to prepare chicken, and the slow cooker does all the work for you. Once cooked, you can use it as-is for simple meals, or add your favorite sauces for variety, like mixing in barbecue sauce for pulled chicken sandwiches, or stirring in salsa for taco meat. Keeping a batch of plain shredded chicken on hand makes it easy to build meals without starting from scratch every time.

2 lbs boneless, skinless chicken breasts (or boneless thighs for extra juiciness)

1 cup low-sodium chicken broth or water

1 teaspoon salt

½ teaspoon pepper (optional, mild flavor)

½ teaspoon garlic powder (optional)

1. Place chicken breasts (or thighs) into the slow cooker.
2. Pour chicken broth or water over the top. Sprinkle with salt, and optional pepper and garlic powder.
3. Cover with lid and cook on low for 6–7 hours, or high for 3–4 hours, until chicken is fully cooked and tender (internal temp 165°F).
4. Remove chicken and shred using two forks. The meat should pull apart easily.
5. Return shredded chicken to the slow cooker, stir to coat in juices, and keep warm until ready to serve.
6. If you don't like your chicken too juicy, strain out some of the cooking liquid before serving.

GROUND CHICKEN PATTIES

Spoon Rating: 🍴🍴🍴
Makes: 4 servings
Texture: Firm outside, tender inside
Temperature: Hot
Prep Time: 15 minutes
Calories per serving: ~250–300
Sensory Notes: Mild, soft bite, simple and consistent flavor

Ground chicken patties are simple, versatile, and great for when you want something easy but filling. You can serve them on a burger bun with your favorite toppings, or enjoy them on their own with a side of vegetables or rice. This recipe also works well if you want to swap the chicken for ground turkey, which has a very similar texture and mild flavor.

1 lb ground chicken (or turkey)

½ cup plain breadcrumbs

1 egg

1 teaspoon salt

½ teaspoon pepper (optional, mild flavor)

½ teaspoon garlic powder (optional, mild flavor)

½ teaspoon onion powder (optional, mild flavor)

1 tablespoon olive oil or neutral oil (for cooking)

1. In a large bowl, combine ground chicken, breadcrumbs, egg, salt, and any optional seasonings. Mix gently (use a fork or gloved hands to avoid touching the raw meat) until combined (avoid overmixing so patties stay tender).
2. Divide mixture into 4-5 equal portions and shape into patties about ½ inch thick.
3. Heat oil in a large skillet over medium heat.
4. Place patties in the skillet and cook for 4–5 minutes per side, until golden brown and fully cooked (internal temp 165°F). If patties are thicker, cook for 6-7 per side. Always use a cooking thermometer for accuracy.
5. Serve hot on burger buns, or plain with sides like mashed potatoes, rice, or steamed veggies.

CHICKEN MEATBALLS

Spoon Rating: 🍴🍴🍴
Makes: 4 servings (about 16 meatballs)
Texture: Tender inside, lightly crisp outside
Temperature: Hot
Prep Time: 20 minutes
Calories per serving: ~280–320
Sensory Notes: Mild, consistent texture, versatile flavor

Chicken meatballs are a lighter twist on the traditional beef version, with a soft, mild flavor that makes them easy to enjoy. You can bake, pan cook, or air fry them depending on what feels easiest. If you don't have ground chicken, you can swap in ground turkey, which has the same texture and cooks up just as well. For a complete meal, try tossing the cooked meatballs with store-bought marinara sauce and serving over pasta: it's quick, comforting, and requires very little effort. These meatballs are also delicious served plain with rice, or even on their own with a dipping sauce.

1 lb ground chicken (or turkey)

½ cup plain breadcrumbs

1 egg

1 teaspoon salt

½ teaspoon pepper (optional, mild flavor)

½ teaspoon garlic powder (optional, mild flavor)

½ teaspoon onion powder (optional, mild flavor)

2 tablespoons grated Parmesan (optional, adds mild richness)

1 tablespoon olive oil or neutral oil (for pan cooking)

1. In a large bowl, gently mix ground chicken (use a fork or gloved hands to avoid touching the raw meat), breadcrumbs, egg, salt, and optional seasonings. Do not overmix, as it can make meatballs tough.
2. Form mixture into 1-inch balls using gloved hands or a small scoop.
3. To bake: preheat oven to 400°F (200°C). Place meatballs on a parchment-lined sheet pan and bake for 18–20 minutes, until fully cooked (internal temp 165°F).
4. To pan cook: heat oil in a skillet over medium heat. Add meatballs and cook for 4–5 minutes per side until browned and cooked through.
5. To air fry: preheat air fryer to 375°F (190°C). Spray basket lightly with cooking spray, arrange meatballs in a single layer, and cook 12–14 minutes, shaking halfway, until golden and cooked through.

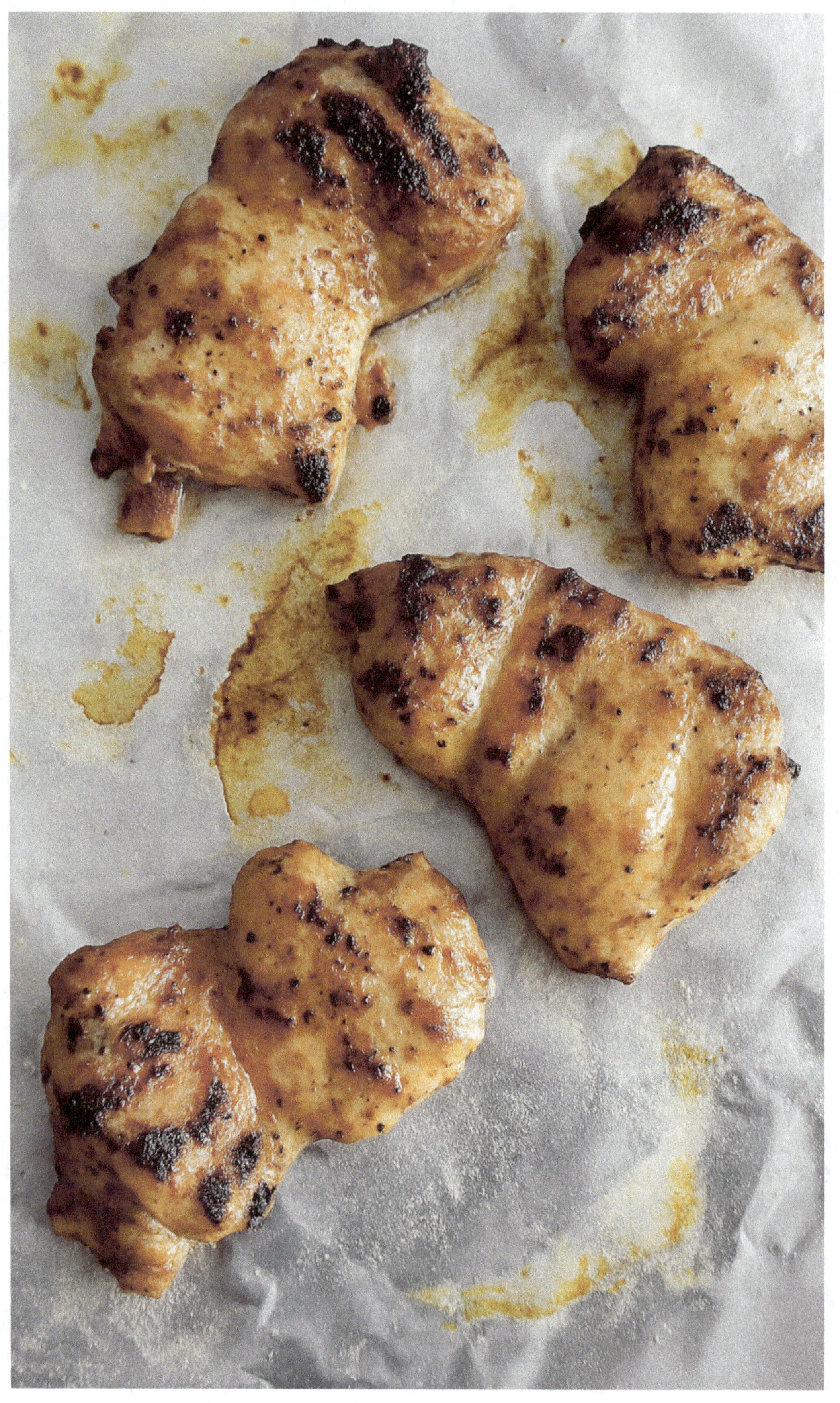

BROILED CHICKEN THIGHS

Spoon Rating: 🥄🥄🥄
Makes: 4 servings
Texture: Juicy inside, lightly crisped outside
Temperature: Hot
Prep Time: 5 minutes
Calories per serving: ~250–300
Sensory Notes: Mild flavor, tender with lightly crisp edges, no bones

Many neurodivergent eaters prefer white meat and dislike dealing with bones, but boneless chicken thighs can be a great option. They stay juicy and tender while developing a flavorful, lightly crisped surface under the broiler. This simple recipe creates reliable results without much fuss, and you can season it mildly or keep it plain to match your preferences. It's great paired with your favorite barbeque sauce, or served plain with a squeeze of lemon over rice or potatoes.

2 lbs chicken thighs (boneless and/or skinless if you prefer)

1 tablespoon olive oil or neutral oil

1 teaspoon salt

½ teaspoon pepper (optional, mild flavor)

½ teaspoon garlic powder (optional, mild flavor)

½ teaspoon paprika (optional, mild flavor)

1. Preheat broiler to high and set oven rack about 6 inches from the heat source. Line a baking sheet with foil for easy cleanup.
2. Pat chicken thighs dry with paper towels. Place on the prepared sheet.
3. Rub thighs with oil and sprinkle evenly with salt and optional seasonings.
4. Broil for 6–7 minutes per side, flipping once, until golden brown and fully cooked (internal temp 165°F).
5. Let rest 3–4 minutes before serving so juices settle and meat stays tender.

BARBECUE BAKED CHICKEN WINGS

Spoon Rating: ⫯⫯⫯
Makes: 3–4 servings
Texture: Sticky outside, tender meat
Temperature: Hot
Prep Time: 15 minutes
Calories per serving: ~350–400
Sensory Notes: Sweet, smoky, tender, with saucy coating

Chicken wings are a classic comfort food, and using store-bought barbecue sauce makes them even easier. Baking instead of frying keeps the prep simple while still giving you tender meat and sticky-sweet flavor. If getting sauce on your fingers is uncomfortable, just use a knife and fork instead of picking them up.

2 lbs chicken wings (split into drumettes and flats, or buy pre-split)

1 tablespoon neutral oil

1 teaspoon salt

½ teaspoon pepper (optional, mild flavor)

1 cup store-bought barbecue sauce

1. Pat wings dry with paper towels. Place them in a bowl and toss with oil, salt, and optional pepper.
2. To bake: preheat oven to 400°F (200°C). Line a baking sheet with foil or parchment. Spread wings in a single layer and bake for 35–40 minutes, flipping halfway, until golden brown and cooked through (internal temp 165°F).
3. To air-fry: preheat to 375°F (190°C). Place wings in a single layer in the basket and cook 20–25 minutes, flipping halfway, until golden and cooked through.
4. Remove wings from oven or air fryer and brush with barbecue sauce. Return to oven for 5 minutes or air fryer for 2–3 minutes to set the glaze.
5. Serve warm with extra barbecue sauce on the side if desired.

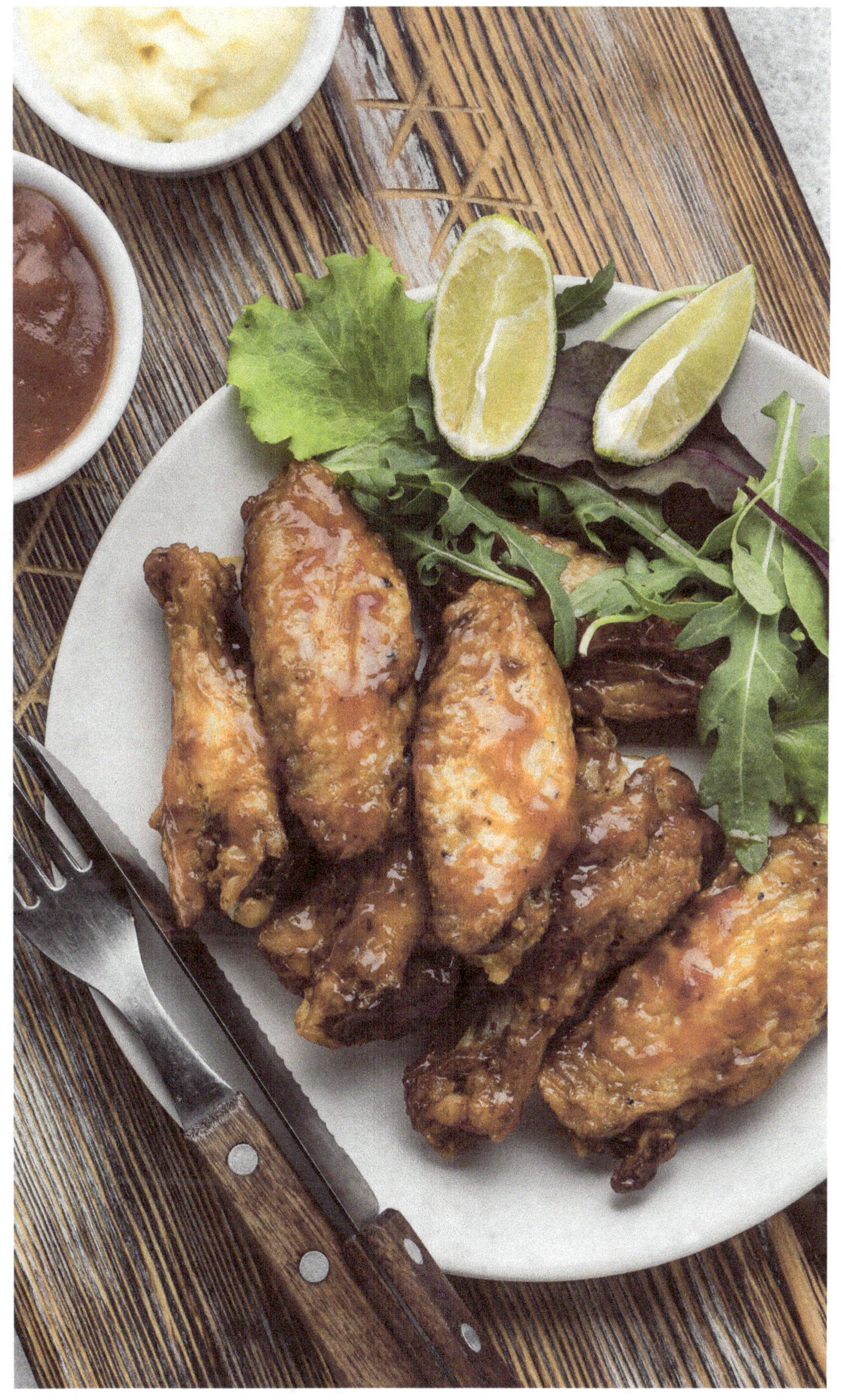

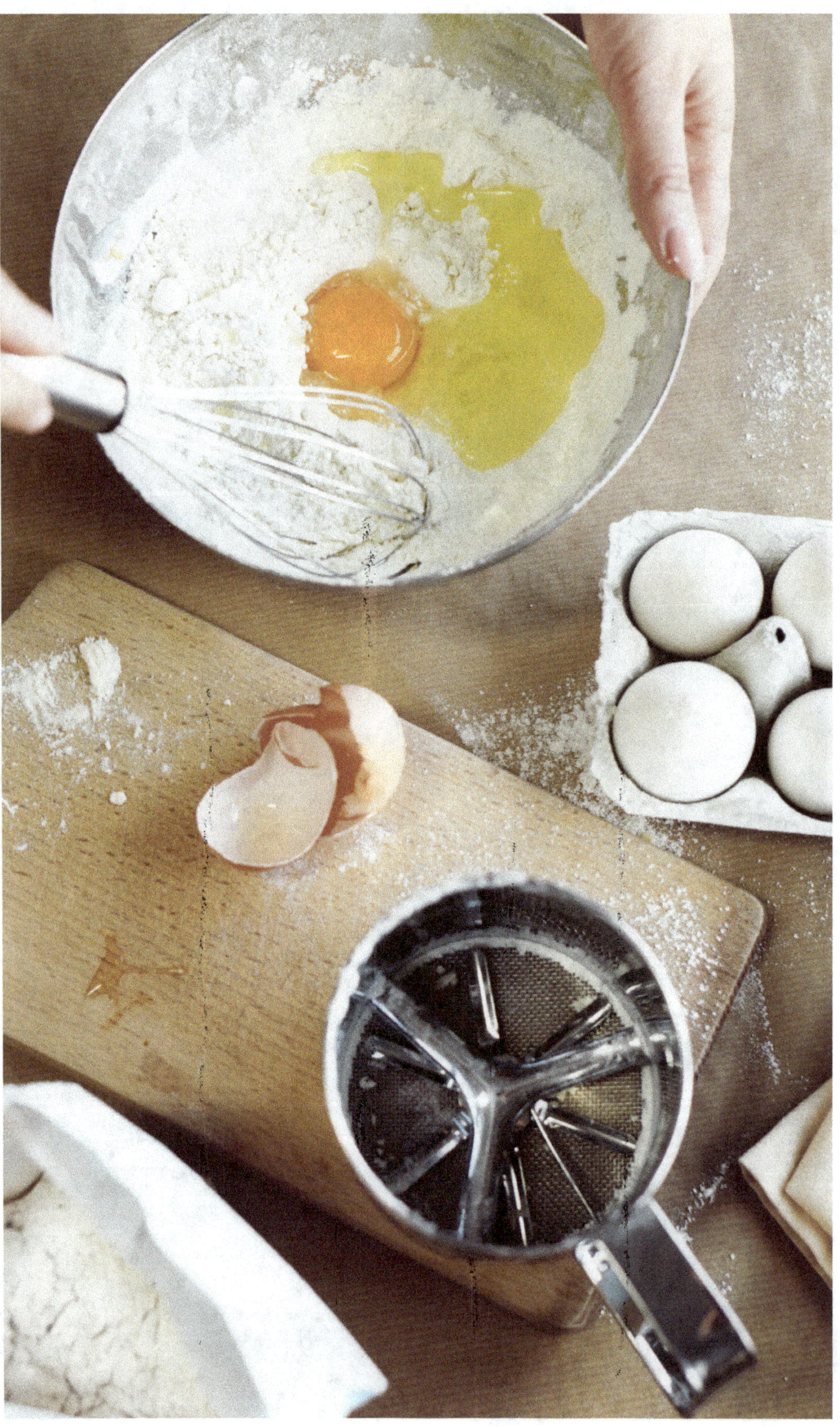

CHAPTER 5: COMFORT FOODS & SWEET REGULATION

Comfort foods play an important role for neurodivergent eaters because they offer stability, predictability, and a sense of calm. The soft textures, warm temperatures, and familiar flavors can help regulate both energy and emotions, especially on days when the world feels overwhelming. Sweet foods in particular are often linked to comfort and reward, making them a natural choice when you need something soothing or grounding.

In this chapter, you'll find recipes designed to highlight that calming effect while also keeping things simple and approachable. From puddings and cookies to warm baked dishes, each recipe emphasizes gentle textures and straightforward preparation. These are foods that feel safe, comforting, and steady. Meals and snacks you can return to again and again when you want familiarity you can trust.

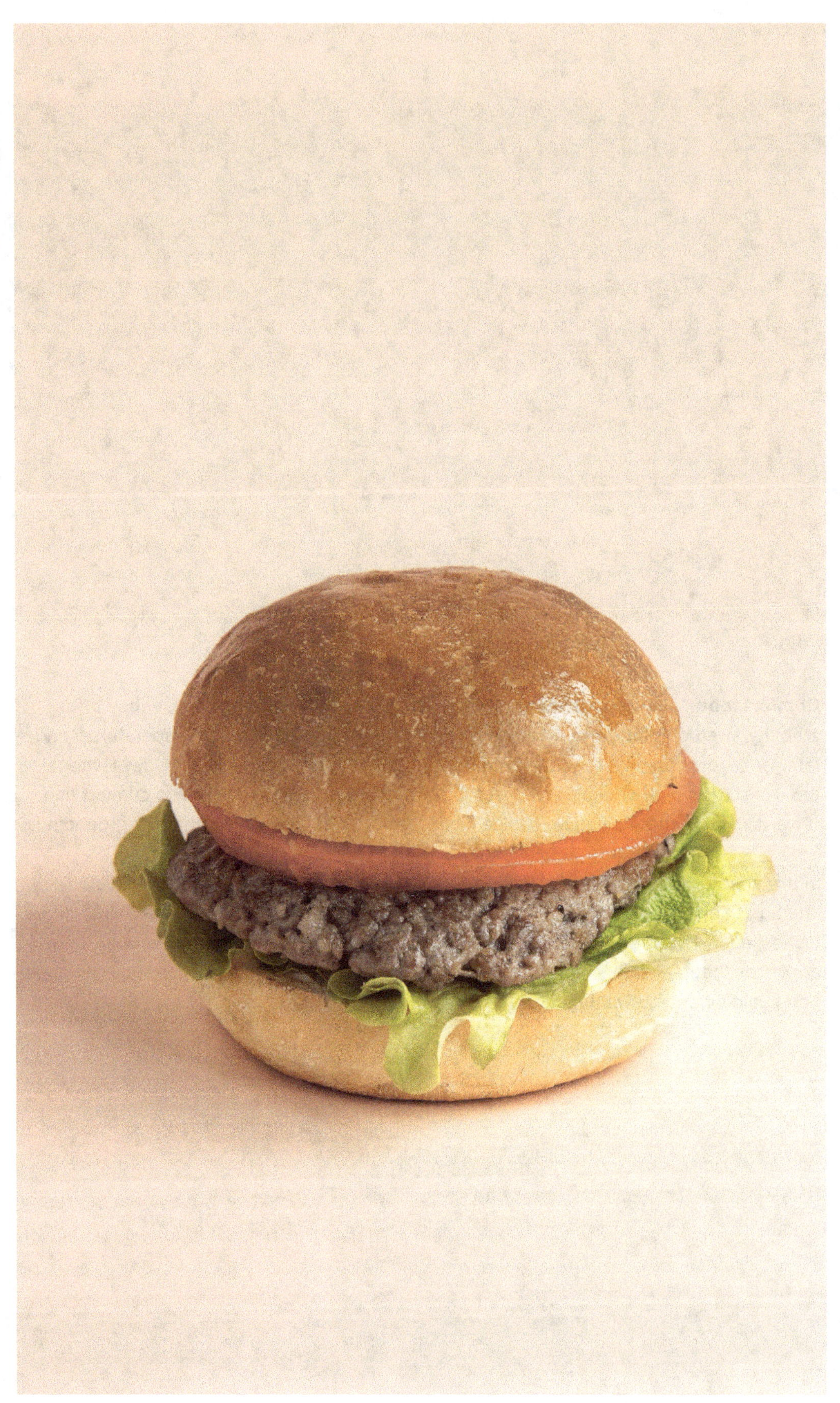

GO-TO HAMBURGER

Spoon Rating: 🥄🥄🥄
Makes: 4 servings
Texture: Tender, juicy patty with a soft bun
Temperature: Hot
Prep Time: 15 minutes
Calories per serving: ~400–450 (without toppings)
Sensory Notes: Soft, mild beef flavor, customizable toppings

A hamburger can be an incredible source of comfort: the smell, the sizzle, and the familiar taste make it a meal many people return to again and again. Using ground sirloin instead of ground chuck keeps the burger flavorful but less greasy, which can make it easier to enjoy if heavier textures are overwhelming. If handling raw meat feels difficult, wearing disposable gloves or using a spoon to shape the patties can make the process more manageable. Great with your favorite toppings and served with pre-made french fries cooked in the oven or air-fryer.

1 lb ground sirloin

1 teaspoon salt

½ teaspoon pepper (optional, mild flavor)

1 teaspoon garlic powder (optional)

4 hamburger buns

Optional toppings: cheese slices, ketchup, mustard, or condiments of choice

1. Place ground sirloin in a mixing bowl. Add salt, pepper, and garlic powder if using. Mix gently with gloved hands or a spoon until just combined.

2. Shape the meat into 4 equal patties about ¾ inch thick, pressing them slightly thinner in the center so they cook evenly.

3. To pan fry: Heat a skillet over medium-high heat. Cook patties for 3–4 minutes per side, or until the internal temperature reaches 160°F (71°C).

4. To grill: Preheat outdoor grill or stovetop grill pan to medium-high heat. Cook patties for 3–4 minutes per side, until fully cooked through.

5. Place burgers on buns and add any toppings you like.

PERFECT BUTTERED PASTA

Spoon Rating: 🍴🍴
Makes: 2 servings
Texture: Soft and silky
Temperature: Warm
Prep Time: 15 minutes
Calories per serving: ~400–450
Sensory Notes: Mild, buttery, consistent texture

Sometimes the simplest foods are the most grounding, and buttered pasta is one of those classics. It's soft, reliable, and comforting without overwhelming flavors or textures. For neurodivergent eaters, it can feel like a safe reset meal: something familiar and easy to prepare when other foods feel too complicated. You can use any shape of pasta you prefer, but small shapes like bowties or elbows can be easier to eat if long noodles feel overwhelming.

8 oz pasta (shells, elbows, or your favorite shape)

3 tablespoons unsalted butter

1½ teaspoon salt

2 tablespoons grated Parmesan (optional, mild flavor)

Freshly ground black pepper (optional, mild flavor)

1. Bring a large pot of water to a boil and add 1 teaspoon salt.
2. Cook pasta according to package directions until tender (usually 8–10 minutes).
3. Drain pasta, reserving a small splash (about 2 tablespoon) of the cooking water.
4. Add butter and ½ teaspoon salt to the hot pasta and stir until fully melted and coating the noodles.
5. Add 1–2 tablespoons of the reserved cooking water if you want a silkier texture.
6. Stir in Parmesan if using. Add pepper only if you enjoy the flavor. It's optional.

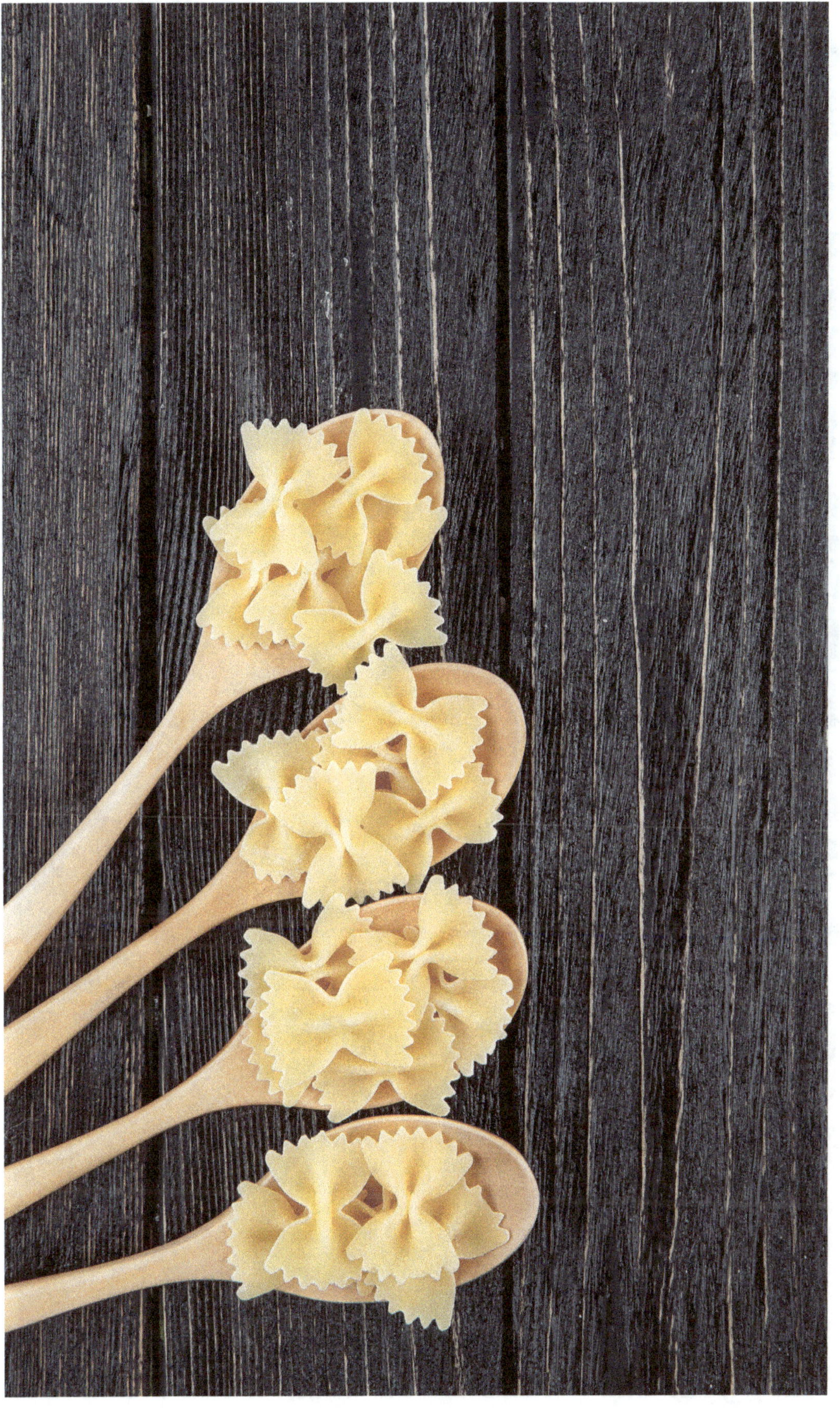

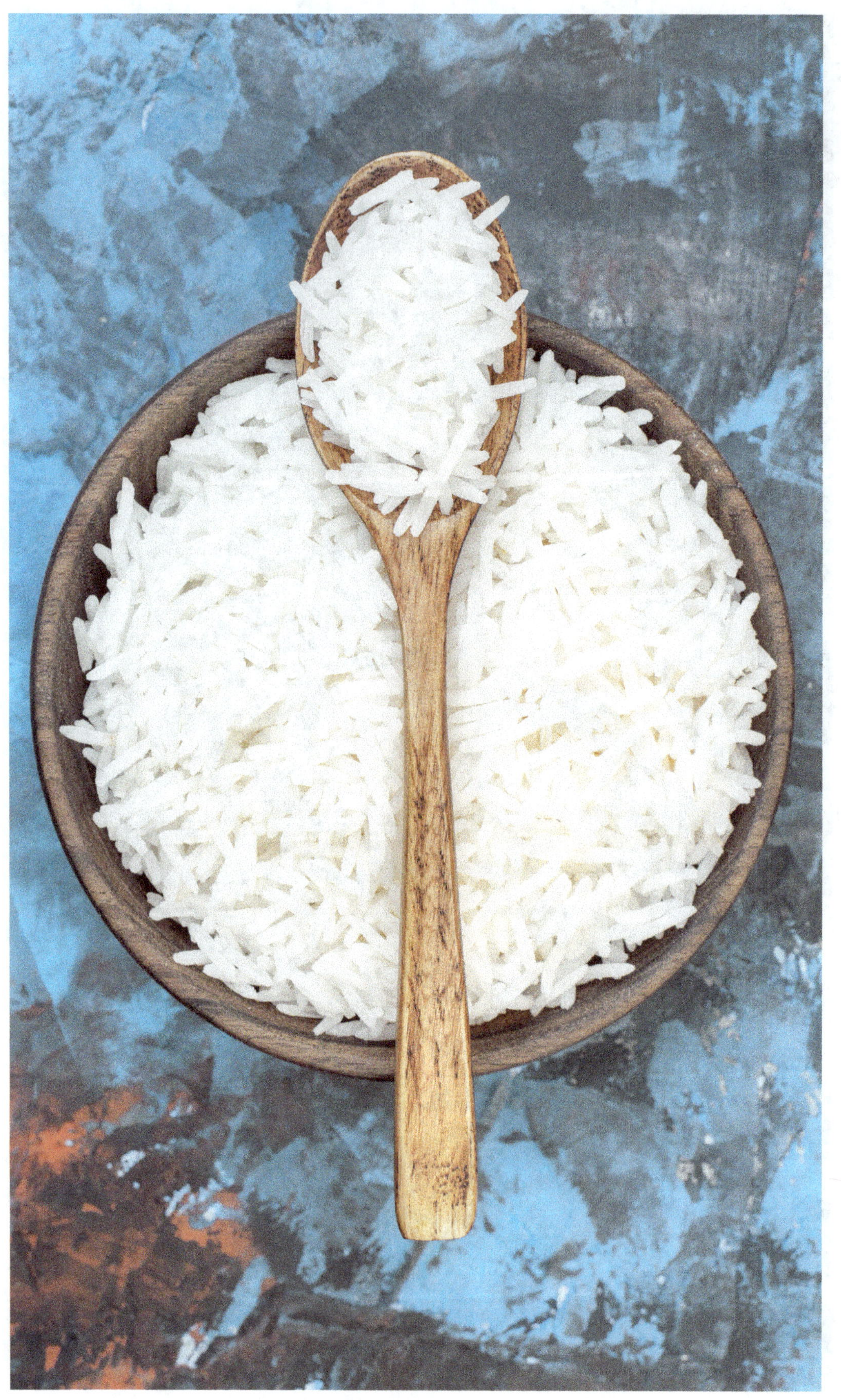

ULTIMATE WHITE RICE

Spoon Rating: ǀ
Makes: 3–4 servings
Texture: Soft and fluffy
Temperature: Warm
Prep Time: 5 minutes
Calories per serving: ~200–220
Sensory Notes: Mild, neutral, consistent bite

White rice is one of the most reliable comfort foods: simple, mild, and a perfect base for countless meals. These instructions are specifically for cooking on the stovetop, not in a rice cooker, so you'll get fluffy rice every time without needing any special equipment. For extra richness, you can stir in a little butter and salt once it's finished cooking, but even on its own it's satisfying and versatile.

1 cup long-grain white rice (such as basmati or jasmine)

2 cups water

½ teaspoon salt

1. Rinse rice under cold water until the water runs mostly clear. This removes excess starch and prevents clumping.
2. In a medium saucepan, bring 2 cups water to a boil.
3. Add the rice and salt, then stir once to combine.
4. Reduce heat to very low, cover tightly with a lid, and simmer for 10–15 minutes without stirring until water is mostly evaporated.
5. Turn off the heat and let the pot sit, covered, for 5 minutes to finish steaming.
6. Fluff rice gently with a fork before serving.

CINNAMON SUGAR TOAST

Spoon Rating: 🍴🍴

Makes: 1–2 servings

Texture: Soft with slight crunch

Temperature: Warm

Prep Time: 5 minutes

Calories per serving: ~180–220

Sensory Notes: Sweet, mild spice, buttery comfort

Sometimes the simplest recipes are the most comforting. Cinnamon sugar toast is quick, warm, and familiar, and using a soft white bread like brioche makes it especially indulgent. The sweetness of sugar blends with the mild spice of cinnamon for a flavor that feels cozy and predictable. This is a perfect choice when you want something easy that still feels like a treat.

2 slices soft white bread (brioche or similar)

2 tablespoons butter, softened

1 tablespoon granulated sugar

½ teaspoon ground cinnamon

1. In a small bowl, mix sugar and cinnamon together until well combined.
2. Lightly toast the bread to your preferred doneness.
3. Spread butter evenly over the warm toast.
4. Sprinkle or spoon the cinnamon sugar mixture generously on top.
5. Cut into halves or quarters if smaller bites feel easier to eat.

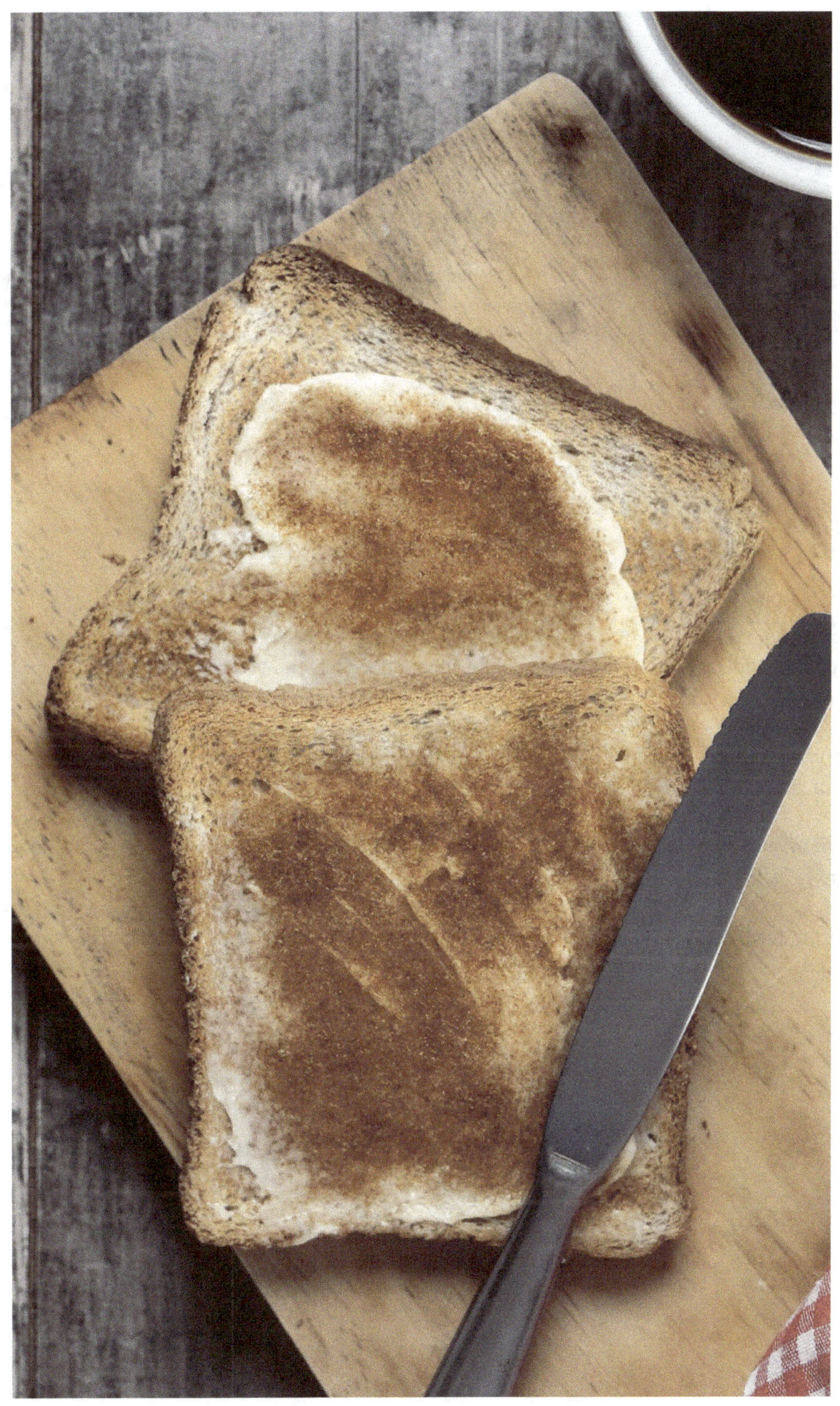

NO LUMPS MASHED POTATOES

Spoon Rating: 🍴🍴🍴
Makes: 4 servings
Texture: Smooth and lump-free
Temperature: Hot
Prep Time: 25 minutes
Calories per serving: ~200–220
Sensory Notes: Mild, buttery, silky consistency

Mashed potatoes are a classic comfort food, but for neurodivergent eaters with texture sensitivities, lumps can make them hard to enjoy. This version uses a hand mixer or stand mixer to whip the potatoes into a perfectly smooth consistency. Adding warm milk gradually helps keep the texture silky, and butter gives extra richness if you want it.

2 lbs russet or Yukon gold potatoes, peeled and cut into chunks

4 tablespoons unsalted butter (optional, for creaminess)

½–¾ cup warm milk (start with less, add more as needed)

1 teaspoon salt (plus more for boiling water)

½ teaspoon pepper (optional, mild flavor)

1. Place peeled potato chunks in a large pot of salted cold water. Bring to a boil, then reduce to a gentle simmer. Cook 15–20 minutes, until potatoes are very tender when pierced with a fork.
2. Drain potatoes well, then transfer to a large mixing bowl.
3. Using a hand mixer or stand mixer fitted with the paddle attachment, beat potatoes on low speed until they begin to break down.
4. Add butter (if using) and mix until melted in. Slowly pour in warm milk, a little at a time, mixing on low until smooth and creamy.
5. Season with salt (and pepper if using). Taste and adjust milk for desired texture.
6. Serve hot with your favorite main dish.

FRENCH TOAST STICKS

Spoon Rating: 🍴🍴🍴
Makes: 2–3 servings
Texture: Soft inside, crisp outside
Temperature: Hot
Prep Time: 15 minutes
Calories per serving: ~280–320
Sensory Notes: Mild flavor, soft but structured, perfect for dipping

French toast sticks are a fun, easy-to-eat version of the classic breakfast dish. Using your favorite white bread works perfectly, but thick brioche slices make them especially rich and soft on the inside with a crisp exterior. Cut into strips, they're ideal for dipping into warm maple syrup.

6 slices white bread (brioche works well), cut into thick strips

2 large eggs

½ cup milk

1 teaspoon vanilla extract

1 teaspoon ground cinnamon (optional)

1 tablespoon butter or coconut oil (for frying)

Maple syrup, for serving

1. Slice bread into 3–4 sticks per slice.
2. In a shallow bowl, whisk together eggs, milk, vanilla, and cinnamon (if using).
3. Heat butter or coconut oil in a large nonstick skillet over medium-low heat until melted and lightly sizzling.
4. Dip each bread stick into the egg mixture, coating lightly but not soaking through.
5. Place coated sticks in a single layer on hot skillet. Cook for 2–3 minutes per side, turning carefully with tongs or a spatula, until golden brown and crisp on the outside.
6. Serve warm with maple syrup for dipping.

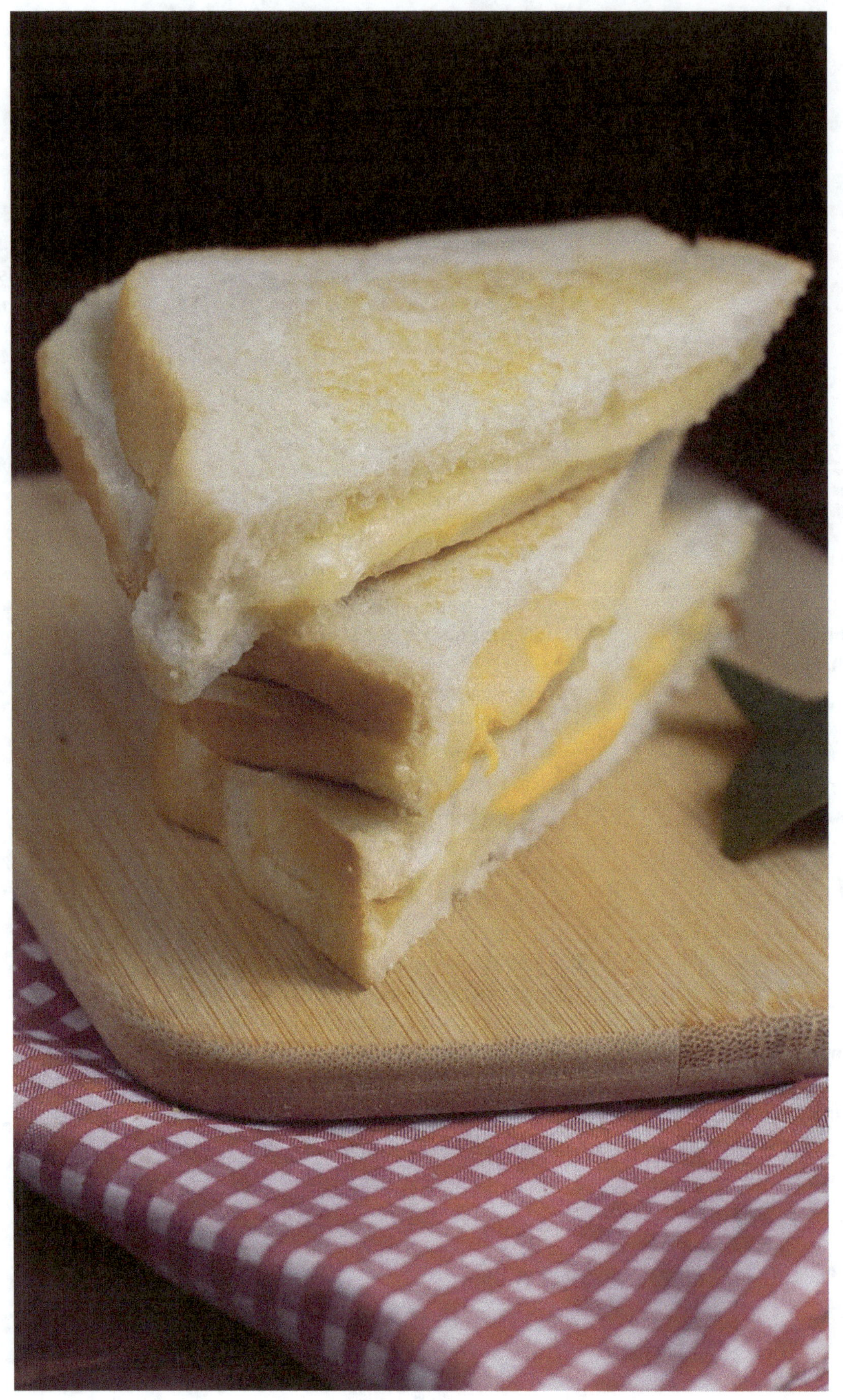

CLASSIC GRILLED CHEESE

Spoon Rating: 🥄🥄
Makes: 1 sandwich (1 serving)
Texture: Crispy outside, gooey inside
Temperature: Hot
Prep Time: 10 minutes
Calories per serving: ~350–400
Sensory Notes: Mild, melty, buttery comfort

Grilled cheese is the ultimate comfort food, simple to make and always reliable. Using your favorite white bread and pre-sliced cheese keeps the process easy and predictable, so you don't have to fuss with shredding or measuring. Cooking on very low heat is the secret to a golden crust and fully melted, gooey cheese without burning the outside.

2 slices of your favorite white bread

2 slices of your favorite pre-sliced cheese (cheddar, American, provolone, or similar)

1–2 tablespoons butter, softened

1. Butter one side of each bread slice evenly.
2. Place one slice, buttered side down, into a nonstick skillet.
3. Add cheese slices on top, then cover with the second piece of bread, buttered side up.
4. Cook over very low heat for 4–5 minutes per side, pressing gently with a spatula, until the bread is golden and the cheese is melted.
5. Cut into halves or quarters for easier handling and serve warm.

BAKED MAC AND CHEESE

Spoon Rating: 🥄🥄🥄
Makes: 6–8 servings
Texture: Creamy pasta with optional crispy topping
Temperature: Warm
Prep Time: 20 minutes
Calories per serving: ~400–450
Sensory Notes: Mild, cheesy, smooth pasta, with optional crunchy top

Baked mac and cheese is the ultimate comfort food. This version is creamy, cheesy, and can be topped with a golden breadcrumb layer for crunch. It's baked in a 9x13-inch casserole dish, making it big enough for family meals or leftovers.

1 lb elbow macaroni

4 tablespoons unsalted butter

¼ cup all-purpose flour

4 cups whole milk

2 cups shredded cheddar cheese

1 cup shredded mozzarella cheese

1 teaspoon salt

½ teaspoon pepper (optional, mild flavor)

½ cup grated parmesan cheese (optional)

1 cup plain breadcrumbs (optional)

1. Cook macaroni in salted boiling water according to package instructions. Drain and set aside.
2. In a large saucepan, melt butter over medium heat. Whisk in flour and cook 1–2 minutes to form a roux.
3. Slowly whisk in milk until smooth. Cook 5–7 minutes, stirring, until sauce thickens.
4. Stir in cheddar and mozzarella on low heat until melted. Add parmesan if using. Season with salt and pepper.
5. Add cooked macaroni to the cheese sauce and mix until fully coated. Pour into a 9x13-inch casserole dish.
6. If using breadcrumbs and parmesan, mix together and sprinkle evenly on top for extra crunch.
7. Bake uncovered at 375°F (190°C) for 25–30 minutes, until the top is golden brown and bubbly. Let rest 5 minutes before serving.

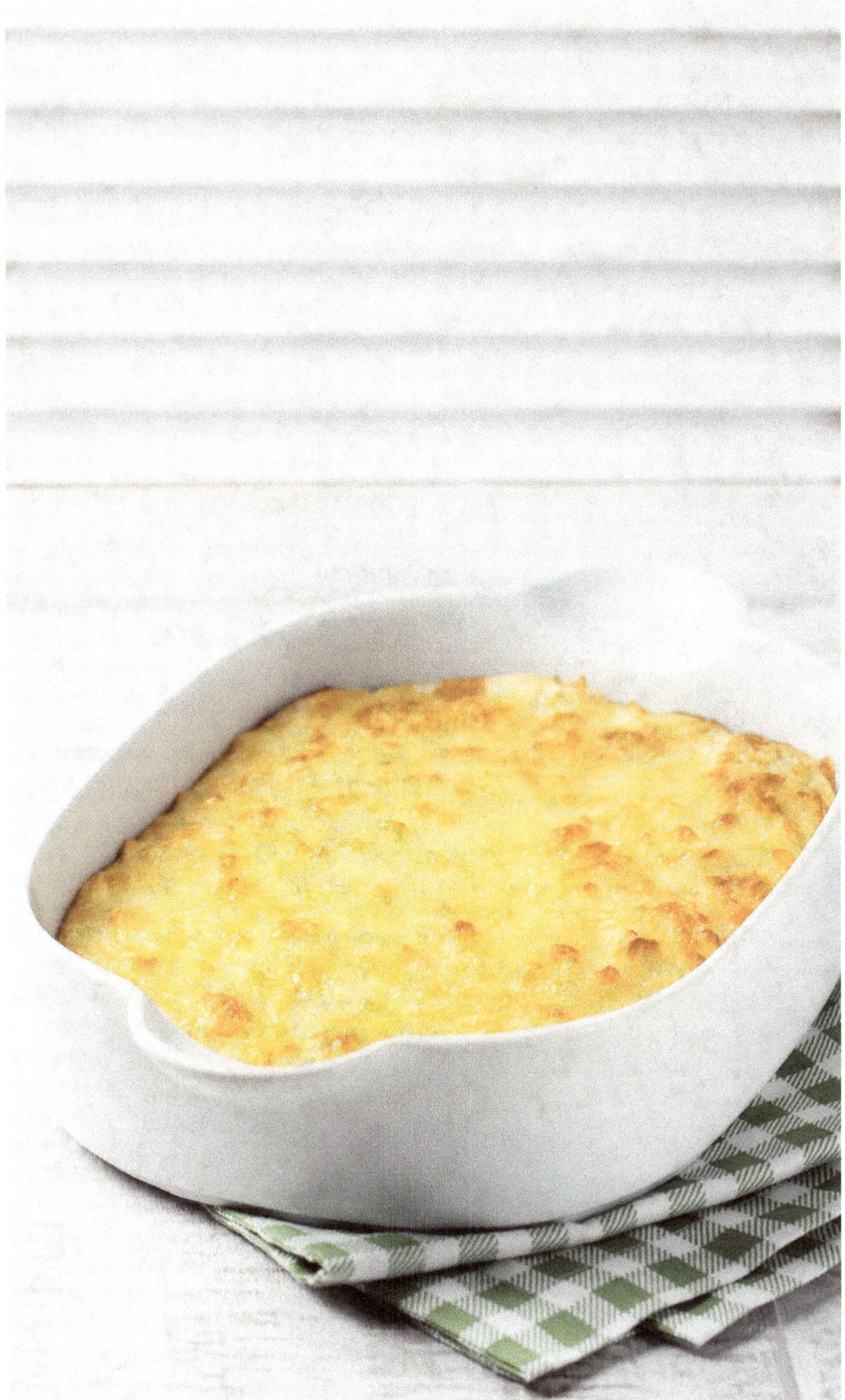

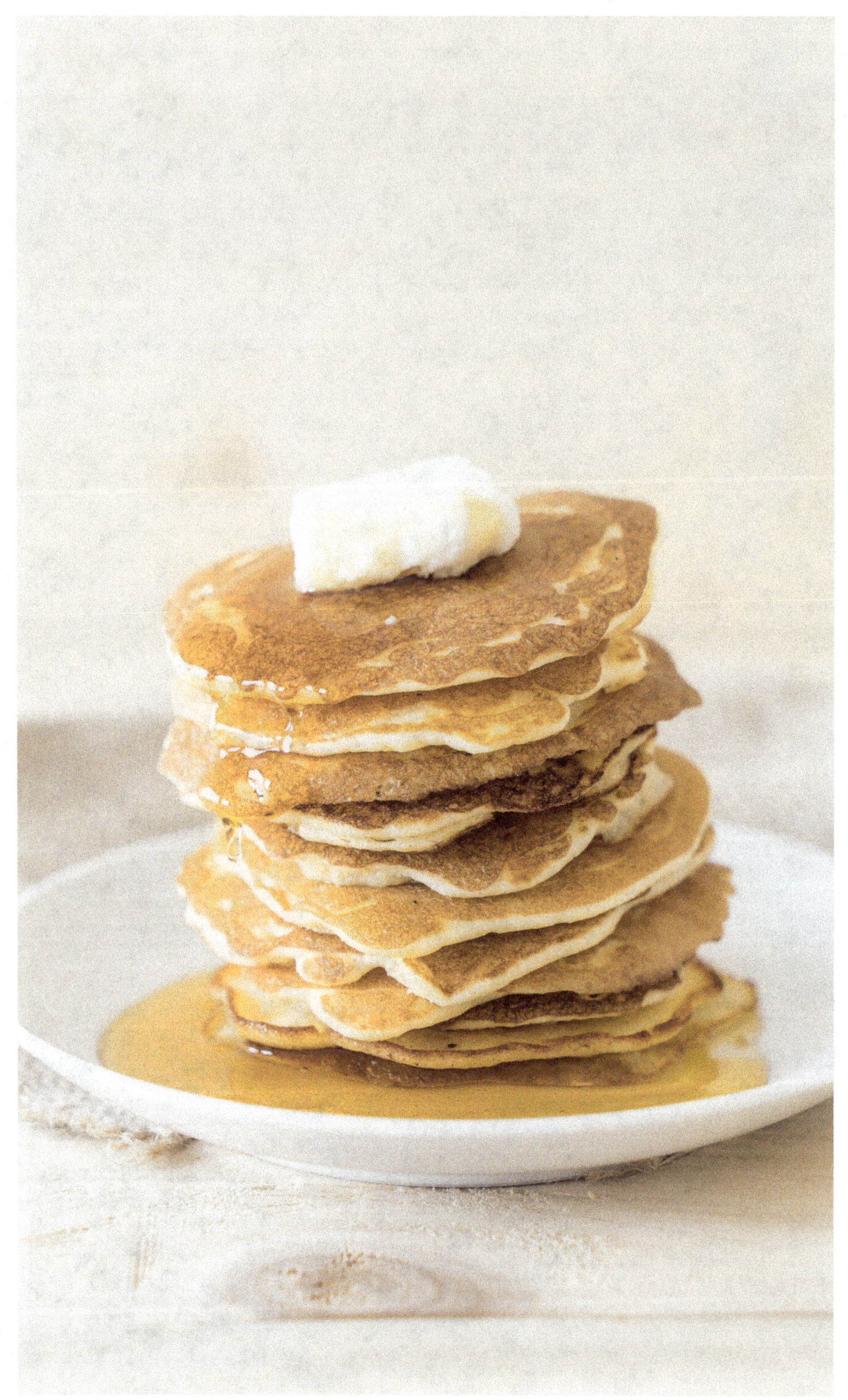

SIMPLE PANCAKES

Spoon Rating: 🍴🍴🍴
Makes: 6–8 small pancakes
Texture: Soft and fluffy
Temperature: Hot
Prep Time: 15 minutes
Calories per serving: ~250–300 (for 2–3 pancakes without toppings)
Sensory Notes: Mild, slightly sweet, soft bite

Pancakes are one of the easiest comfort foods to prepare, and they can be made with just a few pantry staples. The texture is soft and fluffy, and they can be enjoyed plain or with toppings like fruit, maple syrup, or butter. Cooking them in coconut oil instead of butter adds a light sweetness and can be gentler for those who prefer dairy-free options.

1 cup all-purpose flour

2 tablespoons sugar

2 teaspoons baking powder

¼ teaspoon salt

1 cup milk (dairy or non-dairy)

1 egg

1 teaspoon vanilla extract (optional)

2 tablespoons neutral oil, coconut oil or melted butter for frying

2 teaspoons maple syrup (optional)

1. In a mixing bowl, whisk together flour, sugar, baking powder, and salt.
2. In another bowl, whisk milk, egg, oil (or melted butter), and vanilla if using.
3. Pour wet ingredients into the dry mixture and stir gently until just combined. Do not overmix; a few small lumps are fine.
4. Heat a skillet over medium-low heat and lightly grease with coconut oil or butter.
5. Pour about ¼ cup batter per pancake into the skillet. Cook until bubbles form on the surface, about 2–3 minutes, then flip and cook 1–2 minutes more until golden.
6. Serve warm with maple syrup and your favorite toppings.

SOFT CHOCOLATE CHIP COOKIES

Spoon Rating: 🍴🍴🍴🍴
Makes: 12–14 cookies
Texture: Soft, chewy, slightly gooey centers
Temperature: Warm
Prep Time: 20 minutes
Calories per serving: ~200 (per cookie)
Sensory Notes: Sweet, chocolatey, melty softness

These chocolate chip cookies are designed to be soft, chewy, and comforting, perfect for when you need something sweet but not crunchy. Using a bit of cornstarch and slightly underbaking helps create that tender, melt-in-your-mouth texture. They're also easy to make with pantry staples, and you can freeze extra dough balls to bake later for fresh cookies anytime. If aiming for extra chewy, you might chill the dough for 30 minutes before baking (optional, but helps prevent spreading).

1 ½ cups all-purpose flour

½ teaspoon baking soda

2 teaspoons cornstarch

¼ teaspoon salt

½ cup unsalted butter, softened

½ cup brown sugar, packed

¼ cup white sugar

1 large egg

2 teaspoons vanilla extract

1 cup semi-sweet chocolate chips

1. Preheat oven to 350°F (175°C). Line a baking sheet with parchment paper.
2. In a medium bowl, whisk together flour, baking soda, cornstarch, and salt.
3. In a large bowl, cream butter, brown sugar, and white sugar together until light and fluffy.
4. Beat in egg and vanilla until smooth.
5. Gradually mix in dry ingredients until combined.
6. Fold in chocolate chips.
7. Scoop 2–3 tablespoons portions of dough and place on the baking sheet, leaving space between cookies.
8. Bake for 8–10 minutes, until edges are set but centers still look slightly soft.
9. Let cookies cool on the baking sheet for 5 minutes before transferring to a wire rack.

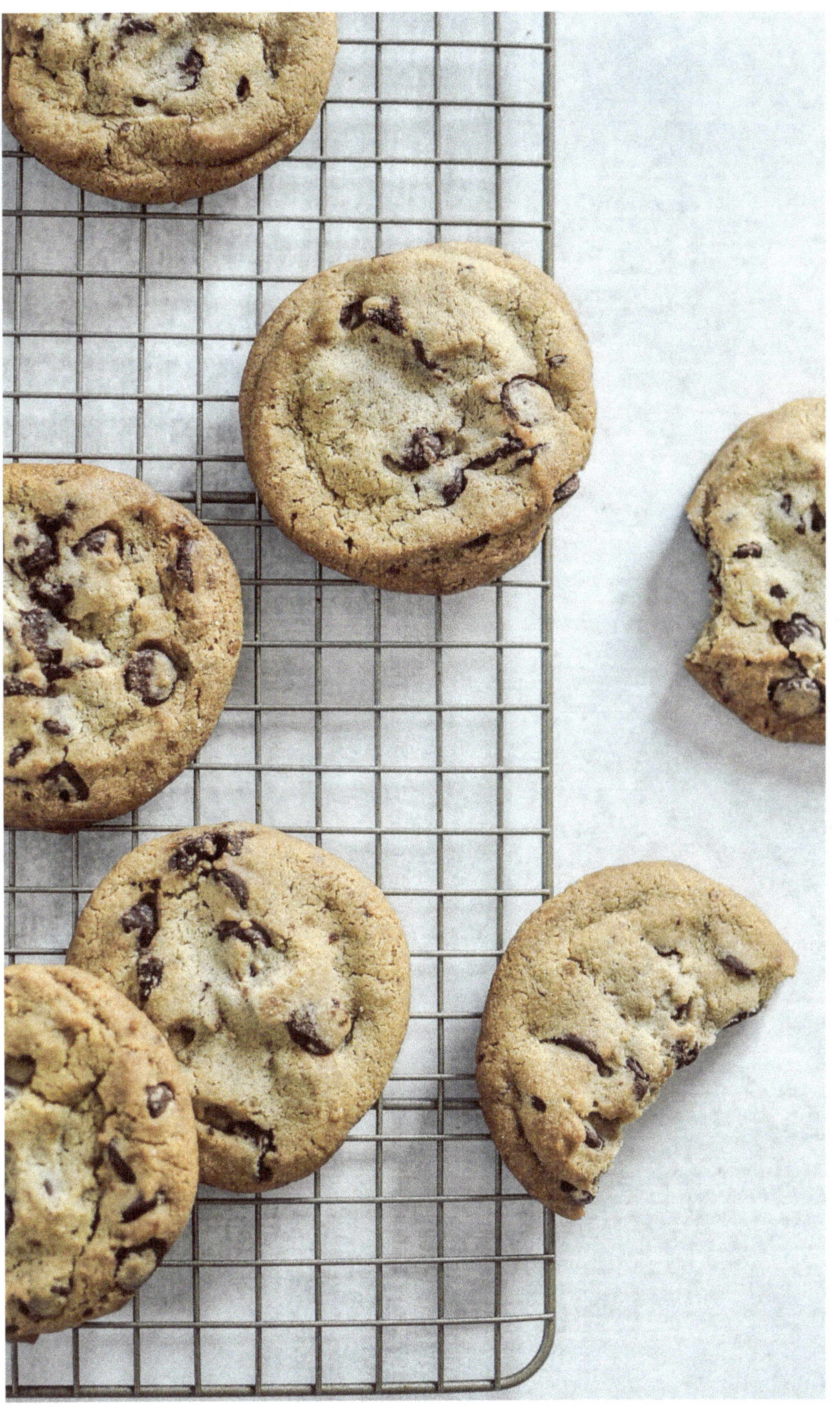

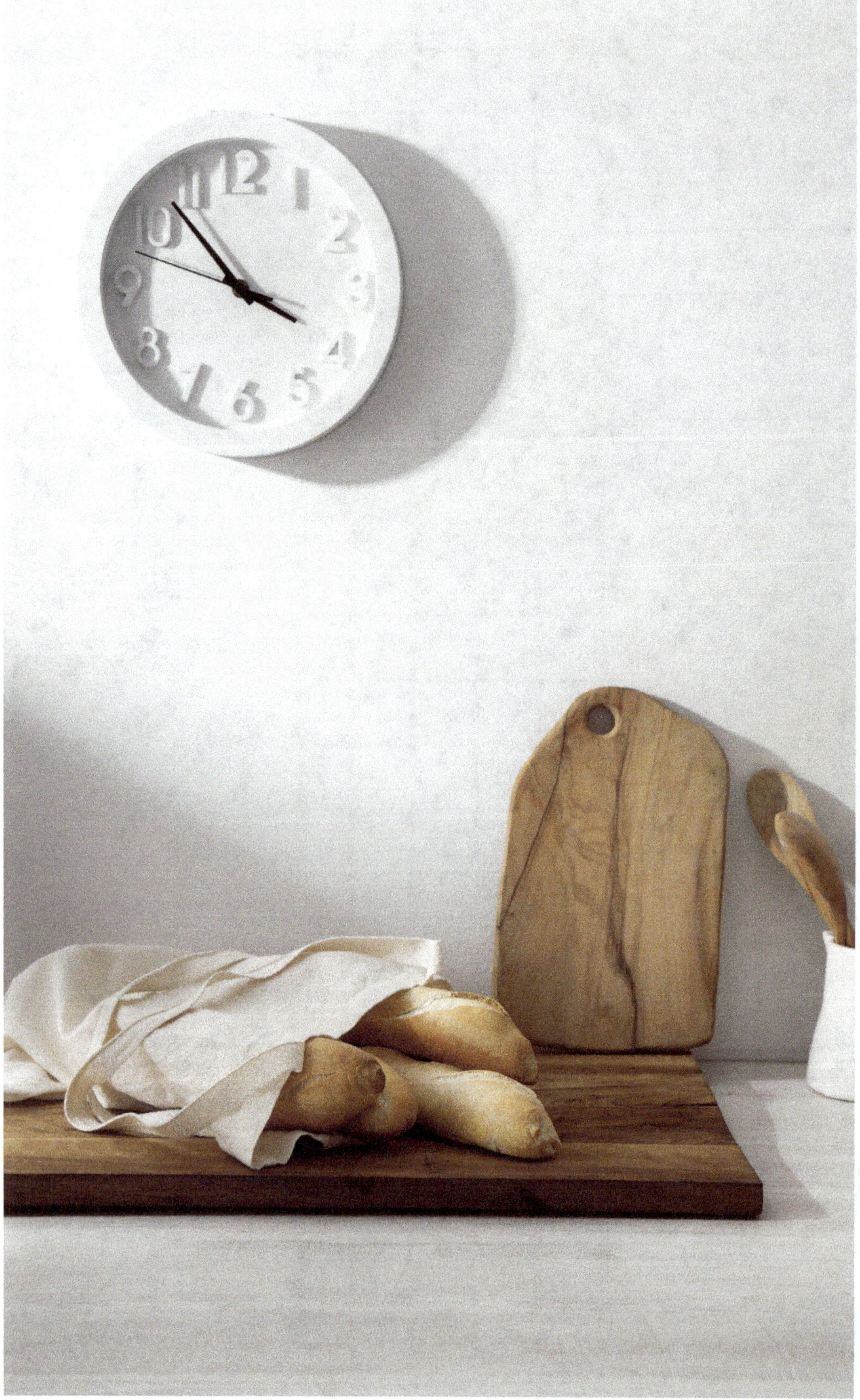

CHAPTER 6: 15 MINUTES OR LESS

Sometimes the hardest part of eating isn't the cooking itself, but the planning, setup, and cleanup. For people dealing with executive dysfunction, even simple meals can feel overwhelming: too many steps, too much energy, too many decisions. That's why this chapter focuses on meals you can get from idea to plate in 15 minutes or less. No complicated prep, no long lists of ingredients, just straightforward recipes that give you the fuel you need without draining the energy you have.

These recipes are built for ease. You'll find simple shortcuts, minimal cleanup, and flavors that are familiar and comforting. Each one can be made quickly with common pantry or freezer items, so there's no need for a big grocery trip or specialized tools. Whether it's breakfast, lunch, dinner, or a snack, these fast meals are about reducing friction and making cooking feel doable again. Even on the hardest days.

3-MINUTE MICROWAVE SCRAMBLED EGGS

Spoon Rating: ⍭⍭
Makes: 1 serving
Texture: Soft and fluffy
Temperature: Hot
Prep Time: 3 minutes
Calories per serving: ~180–200
Sensory Notes: Mild, familiar egg flavor, tender and creamy

Scrambled eggs don't have to mean dirty pans or long prep time. With just a mug, a fork, and a microwave, you can have a warm, protein-rich breakfast in minutes. This method is especially helpful if cooking on the stovetop feels overwhelming or you just need something fast and reliable.

2 large eggs

2 tablespoons milk (or water for lighter texture)

Pinch of salt

1. Crack eggs into a microwave-safe mug or bowl. Add milk and salt.
2. Beat well with a fork until the mixture looks uniform.
3. Microwave on high for 30 seconds, then stir with a fork.
4. Return to microwave and cook in 20–30 second bursts, stirring each time, until eggs are just set (about 1½–2 minutes total).

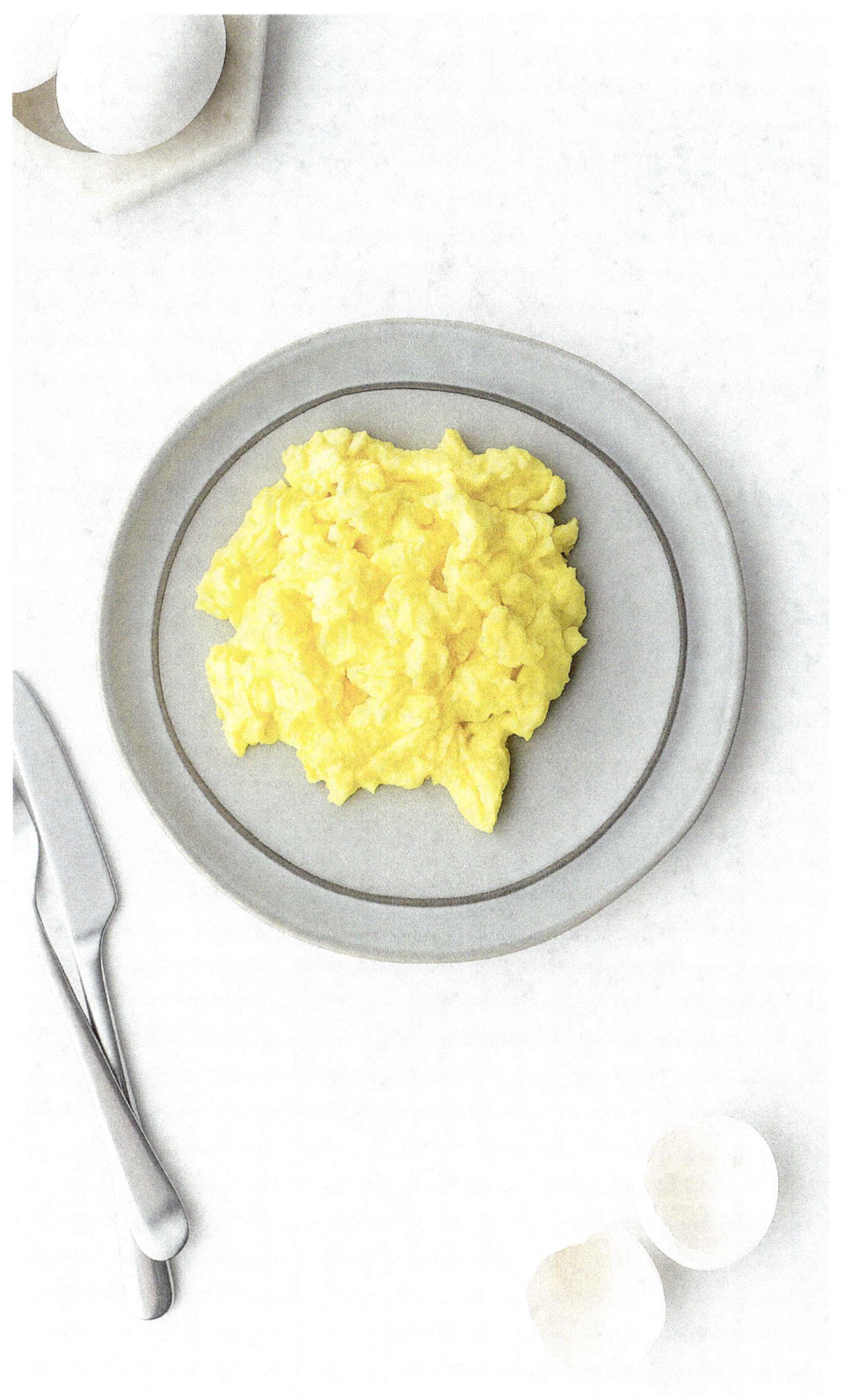

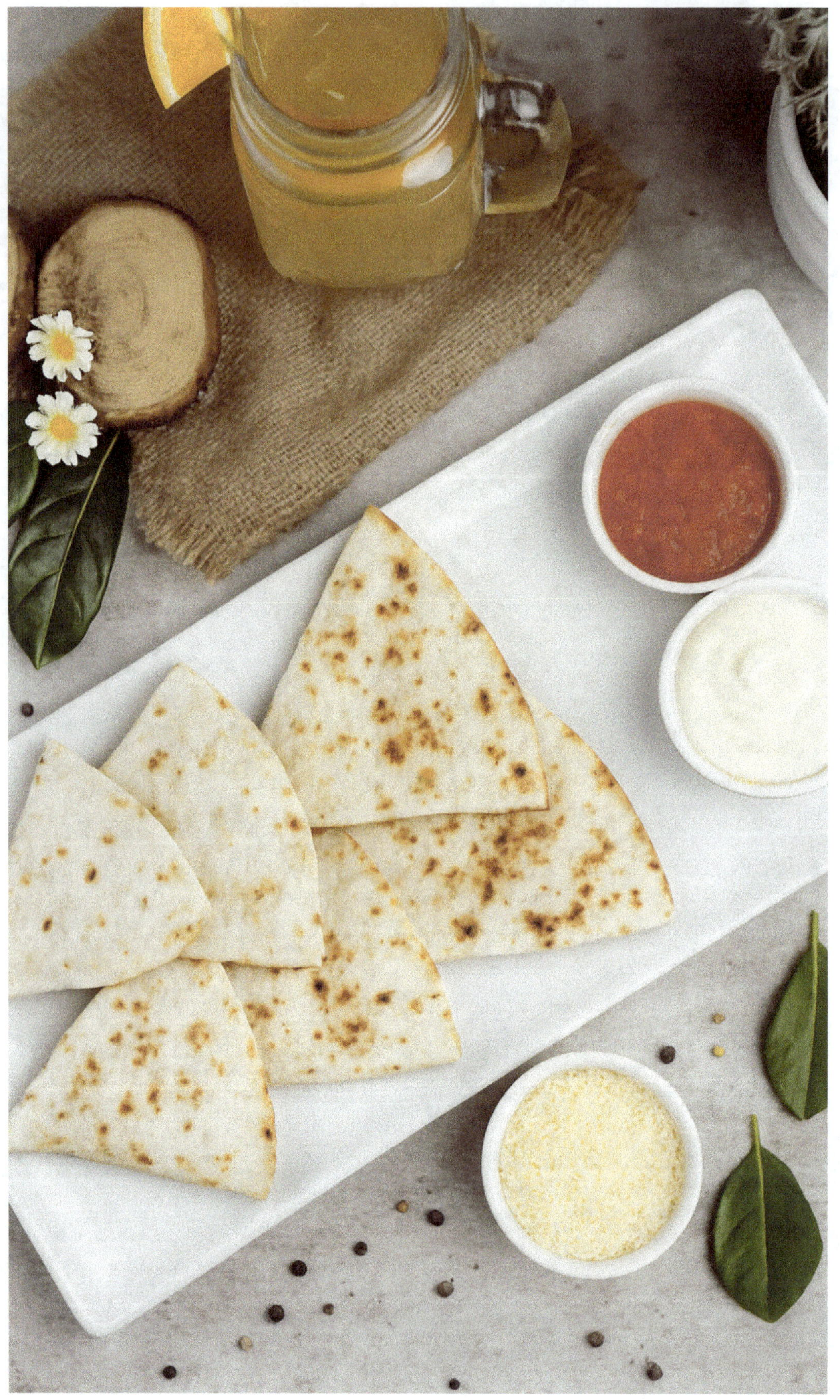

5-MINUTE CHEESE QUESADILLA

Spoon Rating: 🍴🍴
Makes: 1 serving
Texture: Soft inside, lightly crisp outside
Temperature: Hot
Prep Time: 5 minutes
Calories per serving: ~350–400 (without dips)
Sensory Notes: Familiar, melty cheese, mild flavor

A quesadilla is one of the quickest comfort foods you can make: just cheese melted inside a warm tortilla. If you want to boost the protein, you can toss in some pre-cooked shredded chicken or even leftover veggies. It's easy to dip into sour cream or salsa for extra flavor, making this a reliable go-to meal or snack when time and energy are low.

2 medium flour tortillas

½–1 cup shredded cheese (cheddar, mozzarella, or your favorite blend)

½ teaspoon butter or spray oil

Sour cream or salsa, for dipping

1. Place one tortilla on a clean surface and sprinkle evenly with cheese. Add a second tortilla on top.
2. Heat a skillet over medium heat. Add butter or spray oil.
3. Place the tortilla stack in the skillet and cook for 2–3 minutes on one side until golden and cheese begins to melt.
4. Flip carefully and cook another 2 minutes until cheese is fully melted and both sides are lightly crisp.
5. Remove from the skillet, let cool slightly, then cut into wedges.
6. Serve warm with sour cream or salsa for dipping.

INSTANT OATMEAL UPGRADE BOWL

Spoon Rating: 🥄
Makes: 1 serving
Texture: Creamy with soft oats and slight crunch from almonds
Temperature: Warm
Prep Time: 5 minutes
Calories per serving: ~300–350
Sensory Notes: Mild sweetness, nutty crunch, smooth and creamy balance

Sometimes you need a warm meal that comes together in just minutes but still feels nourishing and satisfying. Instant oatmeal is a great base, and with just a few quick upgrades like honey, sliced almonds, and a spoonful of yogurt, it transforms into something more balanced and filling. If you want to add freshness without extra prep, you can keep precut fruit on hand, like berries, melon, or apple slices, that you can toss on top when you're ready to eat.

1 packet (or ½ cup) plain instant oatmeal

¾ cup hot water or warm milk (your choice)

1 tablespoon honey

2 tablespoons sliced almonds

2 tablespoons plain or vanilla yogurt (optional)

½ cup fresh berries, melon or apple slices (optional)

1. Prepare instant oatmeal according to package directions using hot water or warm milk.
2. Stir in honey until evenly mixed.
3. Top with sliced almonds and a spoonful of yogurt.
4. Serve warm.

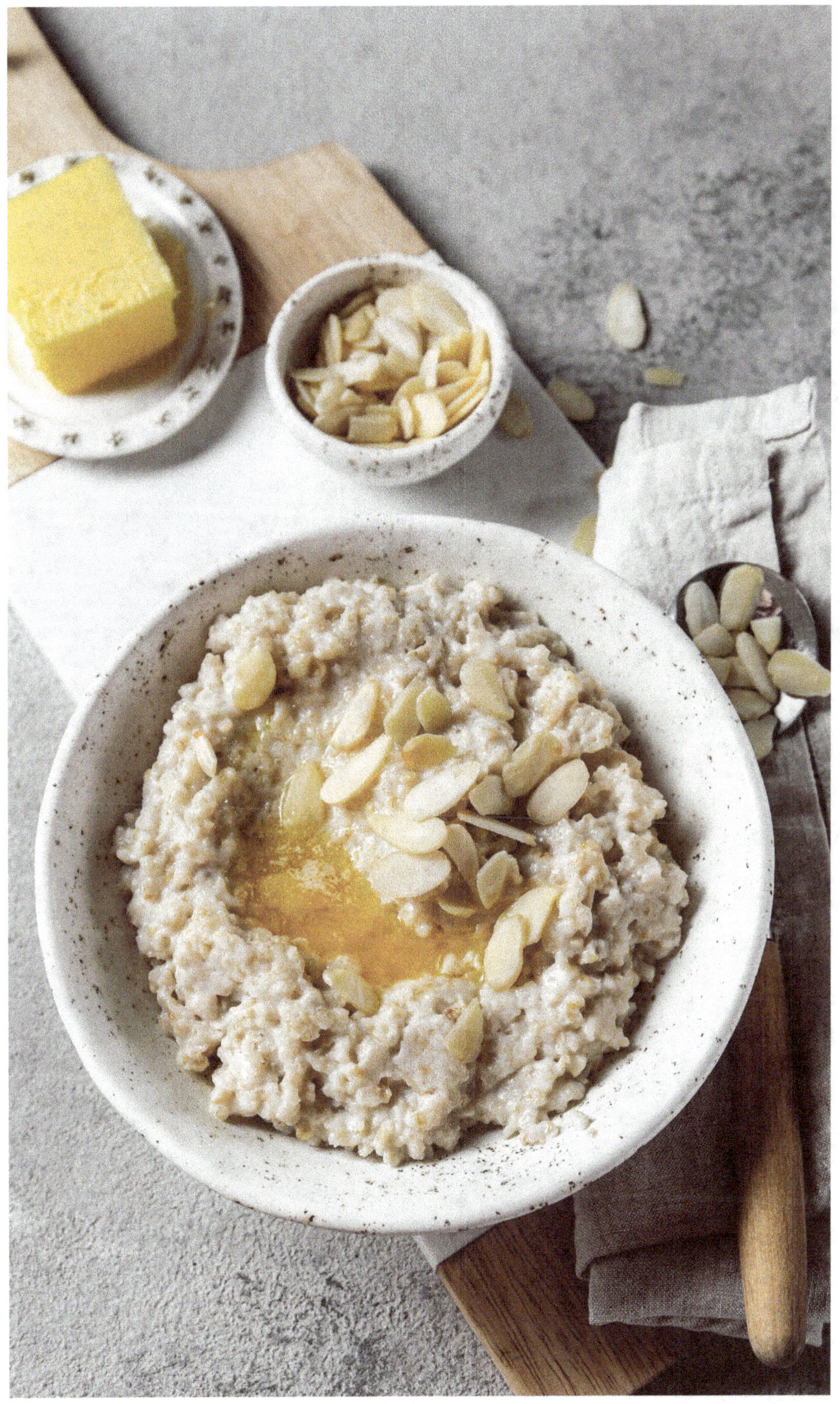

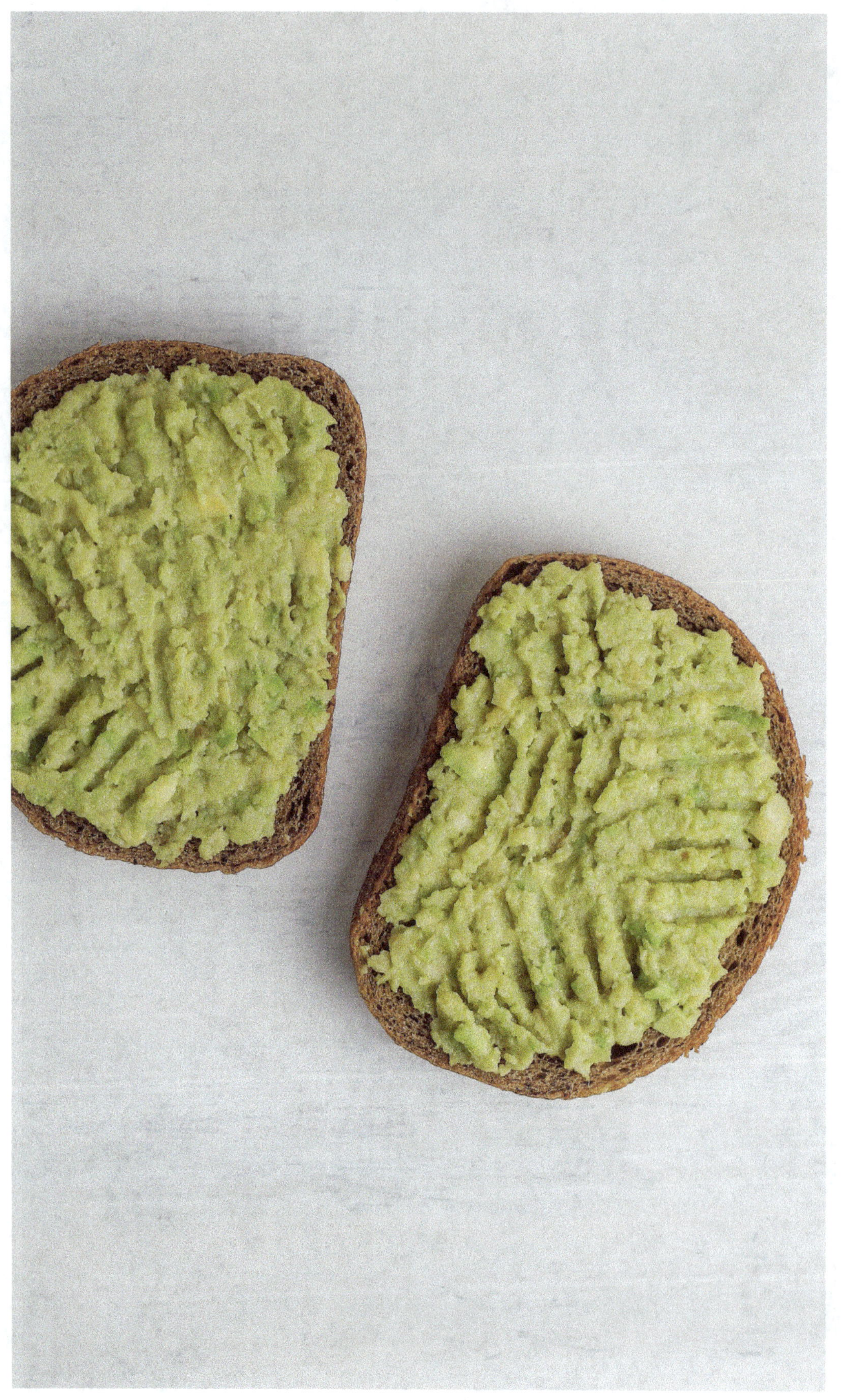

AVOCADO TOAST

Spoon Rating: 🍴
Makes: 1–2 servings
Texture: Creamy topping with crisp toast
Temperature: Room temperature to warm
Prep Time: 5 minutes
Calories per serving: ~250–300
Sensory Notes: Mild flavor, smooth and slightly lemony

Avocado toast is simple, fast, and endlessly adaptable. The creamy mashed avocado makes a satisfying base, and you can boost the protein by topping it with a fried egg, cottage cheese, or even a sprinkle of shredded chicken if you like. Toasting your favorite bread, whether soft white, whole wheat, or hearty sourdough, gives just the right amount of crunch to balance the smooth avocado. The lemon not only adds some brightness to the flavor, but keeps the avocado from turning brown.

1–2 slices of your favorite bread, toasted

1 ripe avocado

Pinch of salt

½ - 1 teaspoon fresh lemon juice

1. Toast bread until lightly golden.
2. Scoop avocado into a small bowl. Mash with a fork until smooth and free from chunks.
3. Mix in salt and lemon juice.
4. Spread avocado mixture evenly over toasted bread.
5. Serve plain, or add optional toppings like a fried egg or cottage cheese.

QUICK TERIYAKI TUNA RICE BOWL

Spoon Rating: 🍴
Makes: 1–2 servings
Texture: Soft rice with flaky tuna
Temperature: Hot
Prep Time: 5 minutes
Calories per serving: ~400–450
Sensory Notes: Mild, slightly sweet-salty flavor, soft and easy to chew

This recipe is as easy as it gets: just mix, heat, and eat. Using pre-cooked rice, canned tuna, and store-bought teriyaki sauce keeps prep under 10 minutes. You can also toss in your favorite veggies, like frozen peas, carrots, or even a handful of precut stir-fry mix, to make it more filling and colorful, or cashew or sliced almonds for crunch.

2 cups pre-cooked rice (store-bought microwaveable packs work well)

1 can tuna, drained

2–3 tablespoons store-bought teriyaki sauce

1. Place cooked rice in a microwave-safe bowl.
2. Add drained tuna and drizzle with teriyaki sauce.
3. Stir to combine, breaking up tuna into small flakes.
4. Microwave on high for 1–2 minutes, until heated through.
5. Mix well and serve as is, or add veggies or nuts if desired.

MICROWAVED LOADED BAKED POTATO

Spoon Rating: ||
Makes: 1 serving
Texture: Fluffy inside, soft skin
Temperature: Hot
Prep Time: 8–10 minutes
Calories per serving: ~400–600 with toppings
Sensory Notes: Neutral potato base, toppings add flavor and texture variety

Baked potatoes don't have to take an hour in the oven: you can get a fluffy, hot potato straight from the microwave in less than 10 minutes. This method is simple and flexible, and once your potato is cooked, you can load it up with your favorite toppings. Try shredded chicken, bacon, cheese, sour cream, or even steamed veggies to make it a full meal.

1 large russet potato, scrubbed clean

1 teaspoon olive oil or butter (optional, for softer skin)

Pinch of salt (optional)

1. Wash the potato and pat dry. Pierce the skin with a fork 4–5 times to allow steam to escape.
2. Place potato on a microwave-safe dish. Rub lightly with olive oil and sprinkle with salt if using.
3. Microwave on high for 5 minutes. Carefully flip and cook an additional 3–6 minutes, until the potato is soft when pierced with a fork.
4. Let rest for 2 minutes before slicing open lengthwise.
5. Fluff the inside with a fork, then add your favorite toppings.

Topping Ideas
Butter and chives
Shredded cheddar or mozzarella
Cooked bacon bits
Sour cream or plain Greek yogurt
Pre-cooked shredded chicken
Salsa or guacamole

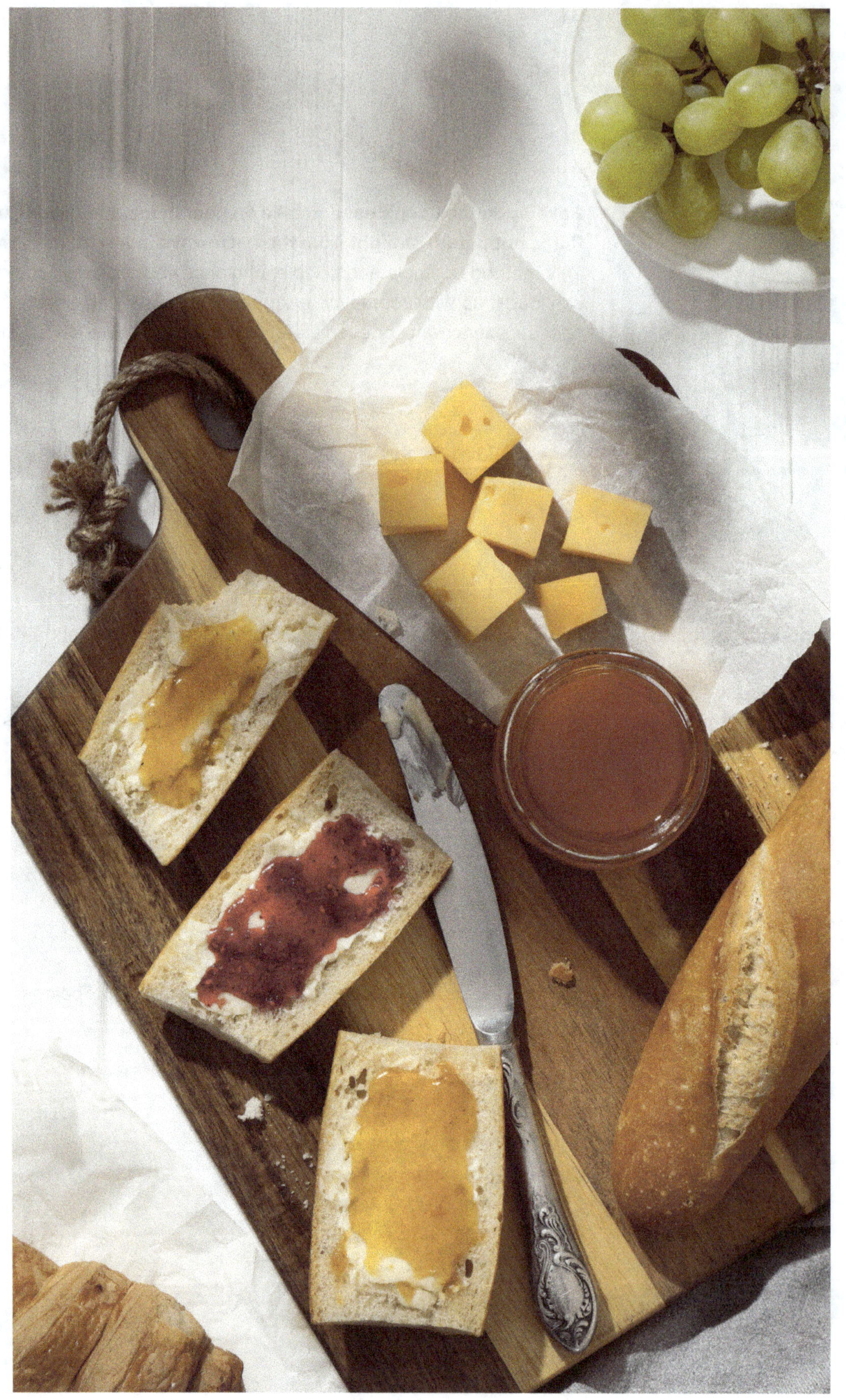

EMERGENCY SNACK PLATE WITH BAGUETTE

Spoon Rating: 🍴🍴
Makes: 2–3 servings
Texture: Crisp outside, soft inside with creamy or savory toppings
Temperature: Warm base, cool toppings
Prep Time: 10 minutes
Calories per serving: ~300–500 (depending on toppings)
Sensory Notes: Warm bread comfort, customizable flavors

Sometimes the best meal is the one that requires almost no cooking at all. A warm baguette from the oven makes the base for an easy "snack plate" that can be built in minutes. It's flexible, filling, and can be tailored to whatever you have on hand, making it perfect for when you're low on energy or decision-making power.

1 baguette, store-bought

Optional toppings and spreads (see ideas below)

1. Preheat oven to 350°F (175°C).
2. Place baguette directly on the oven rack or a baking sheet. Heat for about 5 minutes, until warm and slightly crisp on the outside.
3. Slice into pieces and arrange on a plate with your choice of toppings.

Topping Ideas
Butter, jelly, or honey
Cream cheese or mascarpone
Sliced cheese (cheddar, mozzarella, Swiss)
Store-bought chicken salad or tuna salad
Nut butters (peanut, almond, or sunflower)
Deli meat slices
Fresh fruit (apple slices, grapes, strawberries)

SHUTDOWN DAY SURVIVAL MEAL

Spoon Rating: 🍴🍴
Makes: 1 serving
Texture: Soft noodles with tender add-ins
Temperature: Hot
Prep Time: 10 minutes
Calories per serving: ~400–600 (depending on add-ins)
Sensory Notes: Warm, comforting broth, soft bites

On tough days when cooking feels impossible, instant noodles can be a lifesaver. They're warm, filling, and only need hot water. You can easily upgrade them with simple add-ins that don't require extra cooking, letting the broth do the work for you.

1 pack instant ramen noodles (any flavor)

Water (per package directions)

Optional add-ins (see list below)

1. Cook ramen noodles according to the package directions.
2. While the noodles are cooking, prep any add-ins.
3. Stir in add-ins directly into the hot noodles and broth. The heat of the water will soften vegetables and warm proteins.
4. Serve hot.

Add-In Ideas

Hard-boiled eggs (sliced in half or chopped)
Thinly sliced carrots
Baby spinach or kale
Frozen peas or corn (will thaw in hot broth)
Shredded rotisserie chicken or pre-cooked chicken strips
Tofu cubes
Sliced green onions
Sliced mushrooms

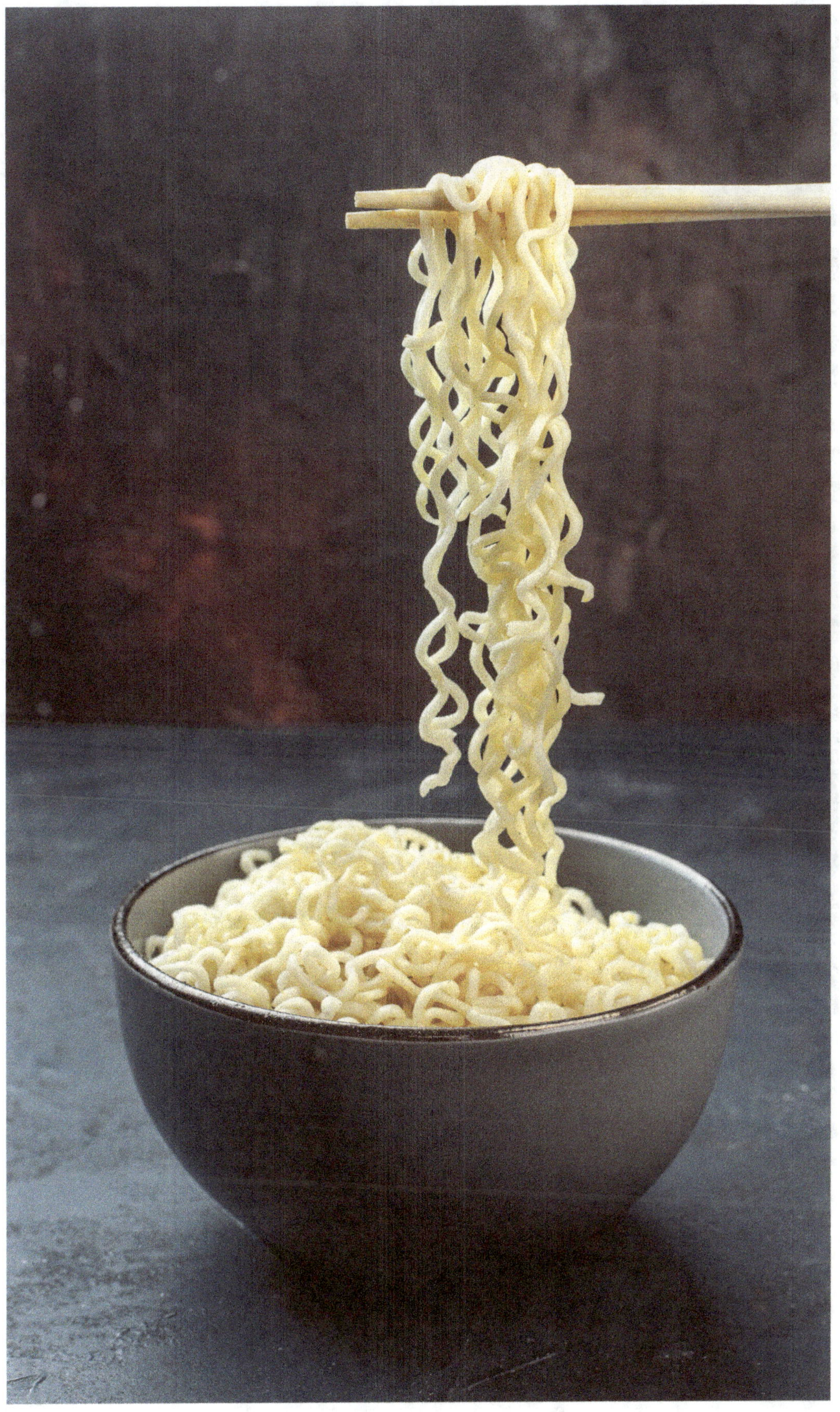

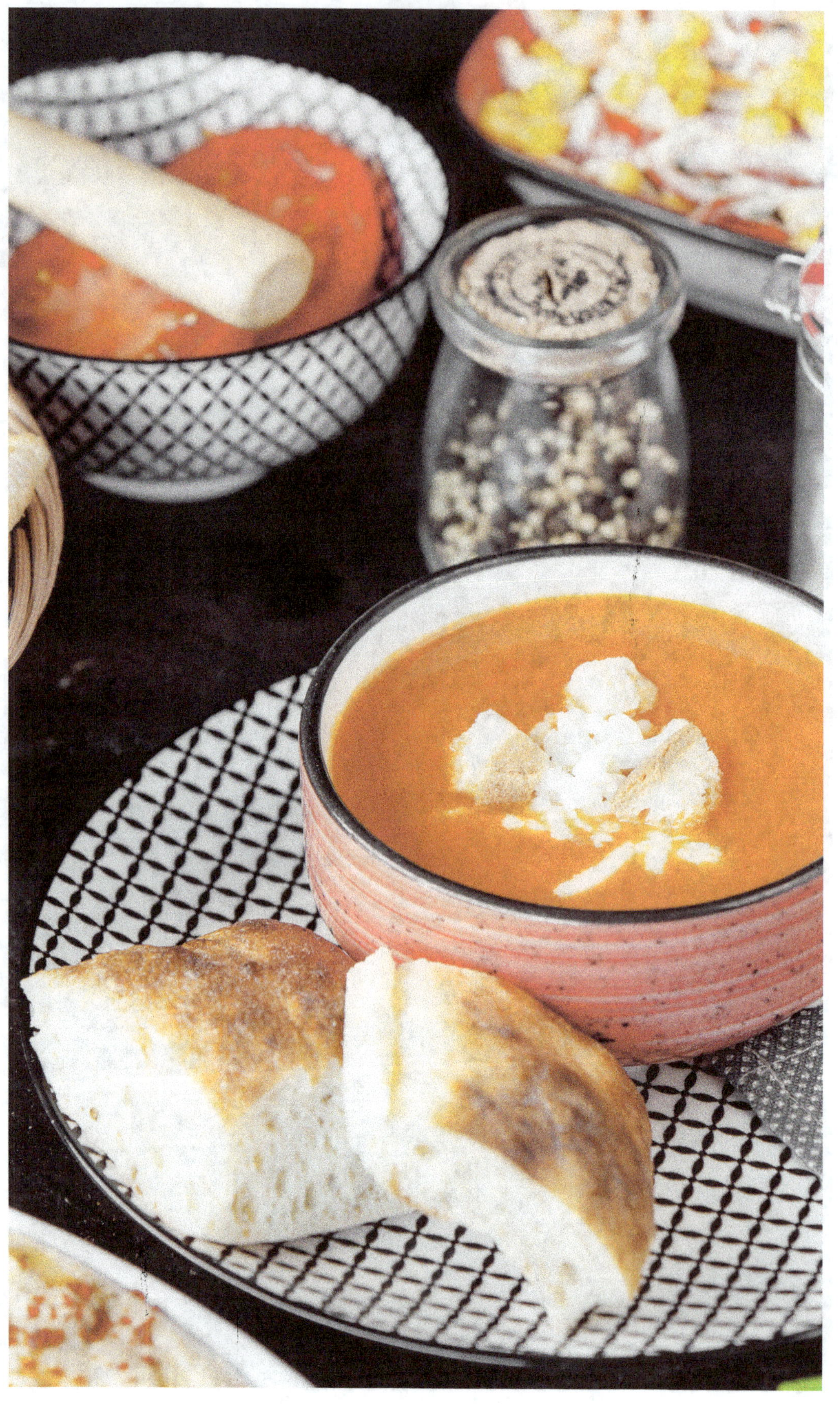

CHAPTER 7: SENSORY CONSIDERATE FOODS

For many neurodivergent eaters, texture is just as important as taste. Some days you may want something crisp and structured like Perfectly Crispy Roasted Potato Wedges or Crunchy Coconut Shrimp, while other times only smooth, gentle foods like Extra Smooth Tomato Soup feel right. This chapter organizes recipes by sensory experience so you can quickly find the texture that works best for you in the moment. Each dish is simple, approachable, and built around consistency.

The key here is variety within safety. A crunchy recipe can provide stimulation and a sense of alertness, while smooth recipes can be soothing and grounding, especially during moments of sensory overload. By understanding which textures feel best at different times, you can choose recipes that help regulate your energy and emotions. These options are easy, adaptable, and mindful of texture sensitivity, giving you tools to enjoy food without stress or second-guessing.

PERFECTLY CRISPY ROASTED POTATO WEDGES

Spoon Rating: 🍴🍴🍴
Makes: 2 servings
Texture: Extra crispy outside, fluffy inside
Temperature: Hot
Prep Time: 10 minutes (plus 10–15 minutes soaking)
Calories per serving: ~200
Sensory Notes: Golden crunch, mild potato flavor, clean bite

Potato wedges are a classic comfort food with a satisfying crunch. Peeling the potatoes gives them a cleaner, smoother bite while still keeping the inside soft and fluffy. Soaking the peeled wedges in cold water before cooking removes starch, which helps them crisp up. You can make these in either the oven or the air fryer. Both give a golden, crispy result.

1 lb russet potatoes (about 2-3 medium), peeled

1 tablespoon olive oil (or neutral oil)

½ teaspoon salt

¼ teaspoon garlic powder (optional)

¼ teaspoon paprika (optional)

1. Peel potatoes, then cut into even wedges: slice each potato in half lengthwise, then cut each half into 3–4 wedges.
2. Place wedges in a bowl of cold water for 10–15 minutes to remove starch. Drain and pat very dry with a clean towel (this step is key for crispiness).
3. Toss wedges in olive oil, salt, and optional seasonings until coated.
4. To bake in oven: Preheat oven to 425°F (220°C). Place wedges on a parchment-lined baking sheet without crowding. Bake 30–35 minutes, flipping halfway, until golden and crisp.
5. To cook in air fryer: Preheat to 400°F (200°C). Arrange wedges in a single layer and cook 12–15 minutes, shaking the basket or flipping halfway, until browned and crunchy.

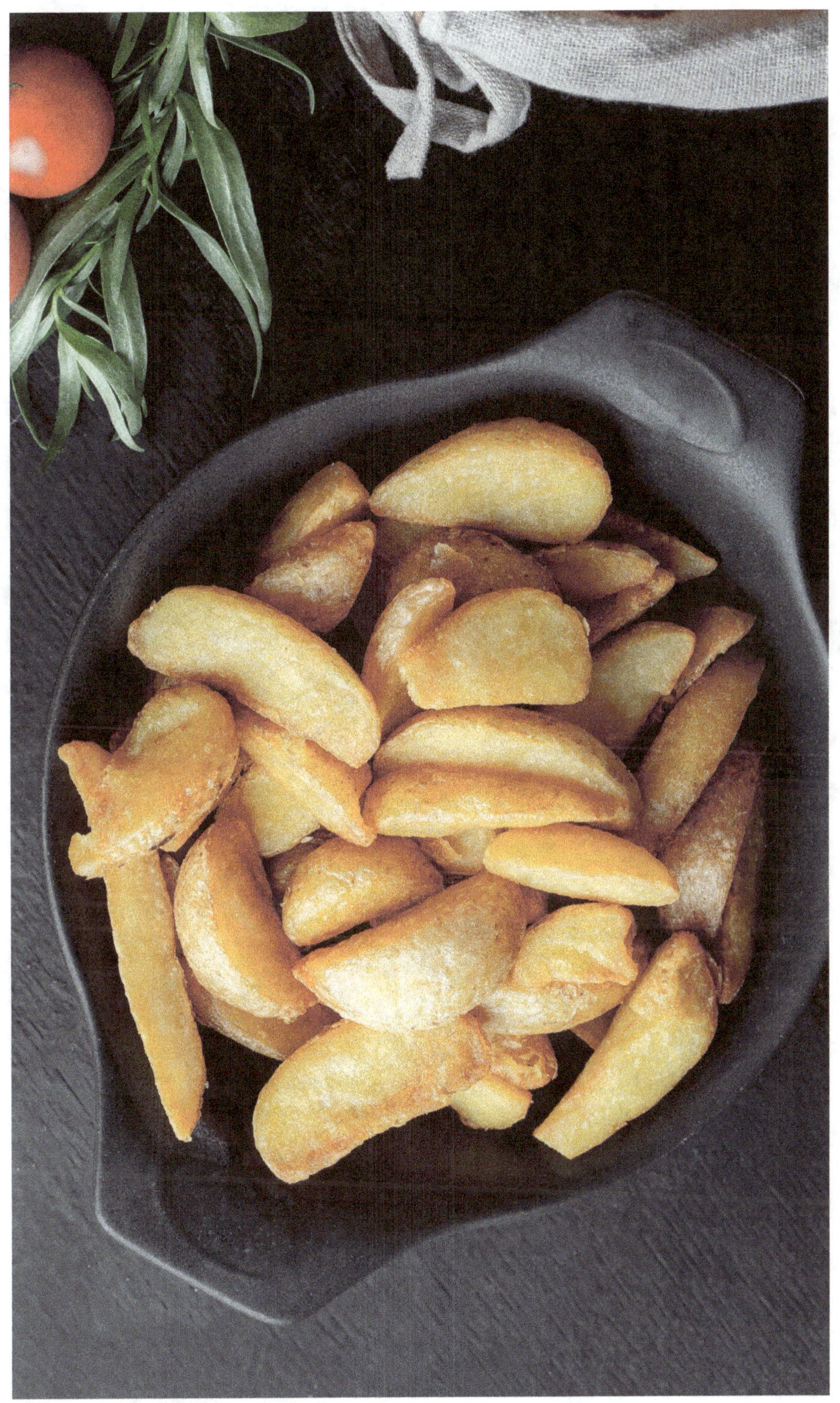

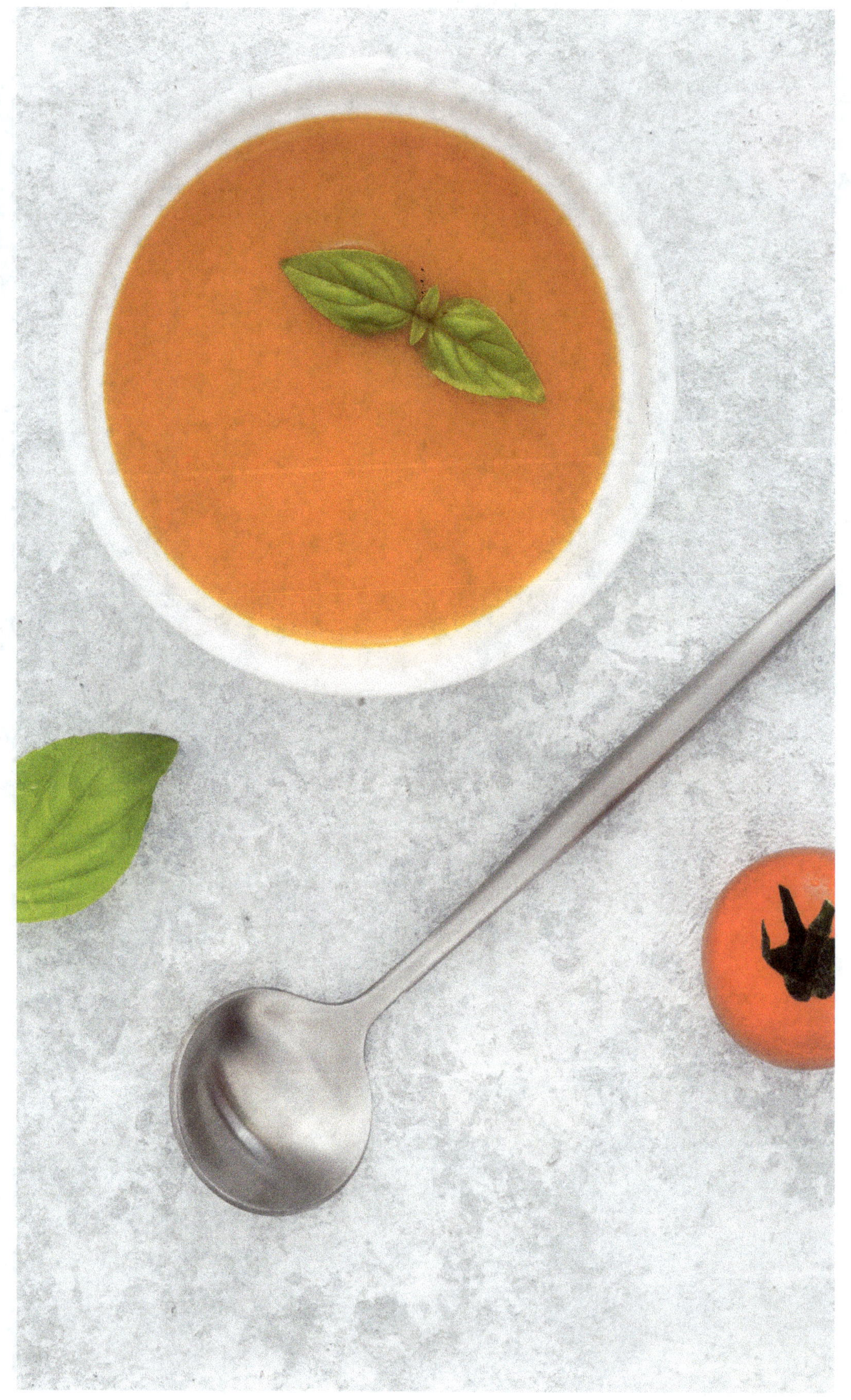

EXTRA SMOOTH TOMATO SOUP

Spoon Rating: 🥄🥄🥄
Makes: 4 servings
Texture: Extra smooth and silky
Temperature: Hot
Prep Time: 10 minutes
Calories per serving: ~180–220
Sensory Notes: Creamy tomato flavor, no chunks, gentle acidity balanced with richness

Tomato soup is one of the most comforting foods, especially when it's silky and smooth with no chunks. Using canned tomatoes makes it easy and reliable, while blending the soup ensures a texture that's gentle and consistent. This version keeps the flavors simple, but you can always pair it with a grilled cheese sandwich for a classic comfort meal.

2 tablespoons butter (or olive oil)

1 small white or yellow onion, chopped

2 garlic cloves, minced

1 (28 oz) can whole peeled tomatoes

2 cups chicken or vegetable broth

1 teaspoon sugar (optional, balances acidity)

Salt to taste

1. Heat butter in a large pot over medium heat. Add onion and cook until soft, about 5 minutes. Add garlic and cook 1 minute more.
2. Add canned tomatoes (with juices), broth, and sugar if using. Stir and bring to a simmer.
3. Simmer uncovered for 15–20 minutes to let flavors meld.
4. Carefully transfer soup to a high-speed blender (or use an immersion blender) and blend until completely smooth.
5. Return soup to pot, warm gently before serving.

CRUNCHY PITA CHIPS WITH EXTRA SMOOTH HUMMUS

Spoon Rating: 🍴🍴🍴
Makes: 3–4 servings
Texture: Crunchy chips, extra smooth dip
Temperature: Chips hot or room temperature, hummus cool
Prep Time: 15 minutes
Calories per serving: ~200–300
Sensory Notes: Satisfying crunch paired with creamy flavor

This recipe combines a satisfying crunch with a silky dip. Baking pita bread into chips gives you a crispy base, while the hummus offers a smooth, protein-rich balance. Store-bought hummus works perfectly if you need a shortcut, or you can make your own and blend it until extra smooth. Together, they make a quick snack or light meal that's easy to prepare and enjoy.

Crunchy Pita Chips

3 pita breads, cut into triangles

2 tablespoons olive oil

½ teaspoon salt

1. Preheat oven to 375°F (190°C).
2. Cut pita into small triangles and spread on a baking sheet.
3. Brush lightly with olive oil and sprinkle with salt.
4. Bake for 8–10 minutes, flipping halfway, until golden and crispy.
5. Remove from oven and cool slightly before serving with hummus.

Extra Smooth Hummus

1 can (15 oz) chickpeas, drained and rinsed

3 tablespoons tahini

2 tablespoons olive oil

2 tablespoons lemon juice

¼ cup cold water (add more for smoothness)

½ teaspoon salt

1. Add chickpeas, tahini, olive oil, lemon juice, and salt to a blender or food processor.
2. Blend until smooth, slowly adding cold water until hummus is extra silky.
3. Taste and adjust seasoning with more lemon juice or salt if needed.
4. Chill before serving with pita chips. Add a drizzle of olive oil to the top of the hummus to keep extra smooth.

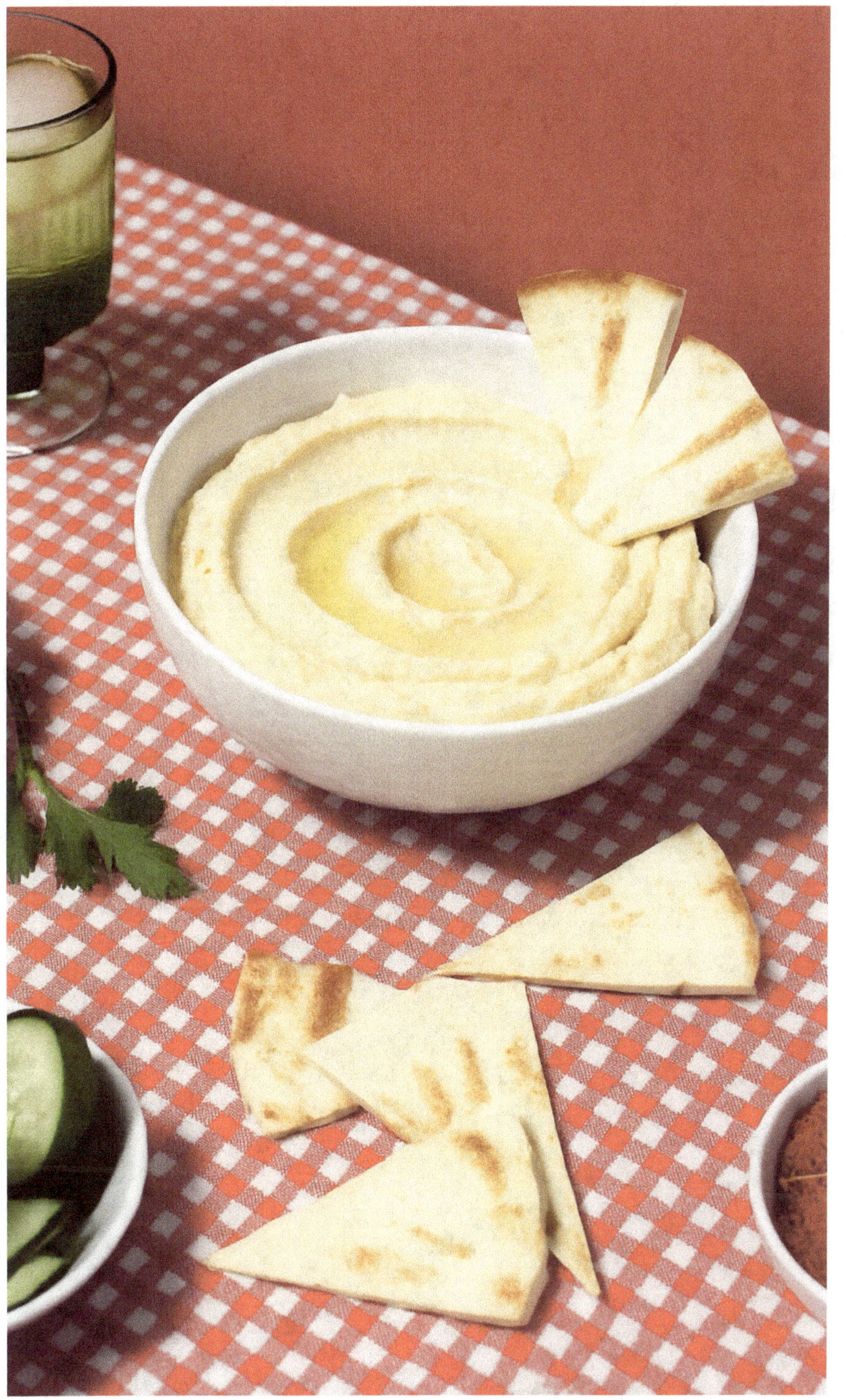

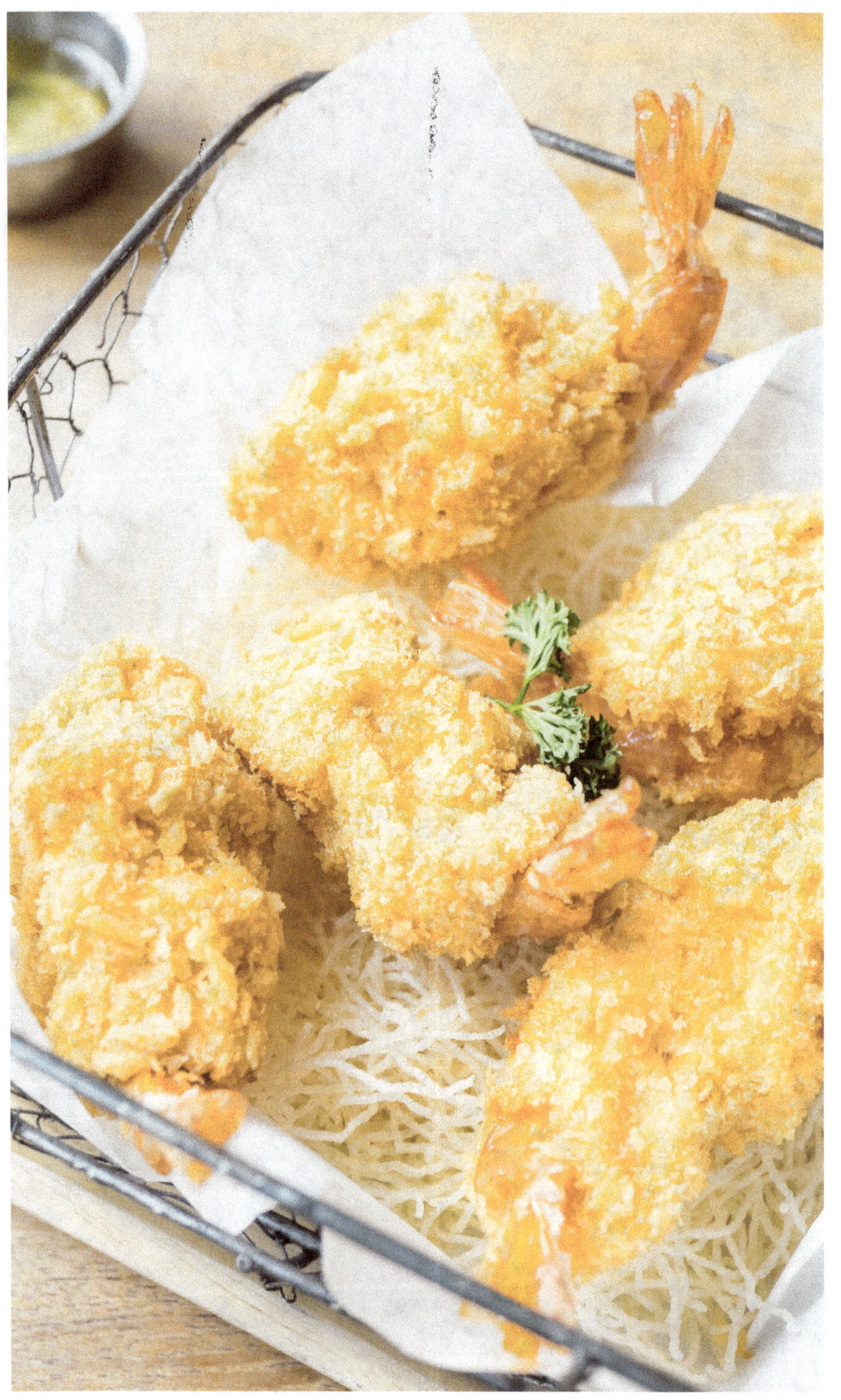

CRUNCHY COCONUT SHRIMP

Spoon Rating: 🥄🥄🥄
Makes: 3–4 servings
Texture: Crunchy outside, tender shrimp inside
Temperature: Hot
Prep Time: 20 minutes
Calories per serving: ~300–350
Sensory Notes: Sweet coconut crunch, mild shrimp flavor, light and crispy bite

Coconut shrimp is crispy, both sweet and salty, fun to eat, and pairs perfectly with dipping sauces. You can keep it simple with cocktail sauce, go sweet with honey mustard or sweet chili sauce, or try creamy ranch for a cool contrast. Buying raw shrimp that's already peeled and deveined makes prep much easier, and you can choose to keep the tails on or off depending on what feels most comfortable. Use gloves or tongs if you don't want to touch the raw shrimp. Cook them in the oven or air fryer for a crunchy coating with tender shrimp inside.

1 lb raw shrimp, peeled and deveined (tail on or off)

½ cup all-purpose flour

2 eggs, beaten

1 cup shredded unsweetened coconut

½ cup plain breadcrumbs

1 teaspoon salt

Cooking spray or 2–3 tablespoons neutral oil

1. If using frozen shrimp, thaw fully in the fridge overnight or under cold running water before starting. Pat shrimp very dry with paper towels.
2. Place flour into a large zip-top bag. Add shrimp, seal, and shake until lightly coated.
3. Set up two more bowls: one with beaten eggs, and one with coconut, breadcrumbs, and salt mixed together.
4. Dip each floured shrimp in the egg, then coat fully in the coconut-breadcrumb mixture.
5. To bake: preheat oven to 400°F (200°C). Place shrimp on a parchment-lined sheet, spray lightly with cooking spray, and bake for 12–15 minutes until golden and cooked through.
6. To air fry: preheat air fryer to 375°F (190°C). Arrange shrimp in a single layer, spray lightly, and cook for 8–10 minutes, flipping halfway.
7. Serve warm with your favorite dipping sauce (cocktail sauce, sweet chili, ranch, or honey mustard all work well).

CRUNCHY CASHEW CHICKEN AND RICE

Spoon Rating: ||||
Makes: 3–4 servings
Texture: Crunchy cashews, tender chicken, soft vegetables
Temperature: Hot
Prep Time: 20 minutes
Calories per serving: ~450–500
Sensory Notes: Sweet-savory sauce, reliable chicken texture, crisp nutty crunch

Cashew chicken is a colorful, comforting dish that combines tender chicken with crunchy roasted cashews and vegetables. Using roasted and salted cashews keeps things simple, while the mix of peppers and onion adds natural sweetness and flavor. You can easily swap in any vegetables you prefer, like broccoli, zucchini, or snap peas, making this a flexible meal that works with whatever you have on hand. Ask your butcher to cut chicken into cubes and handle with gloves or tongs if you don't want to touch the raw chicken.

1 lb boneless, skinless chicken breast, cut into bite-sized cubes

1 red bell pepper, chopped

1 yellow bell pepper, chopped

1 small onion, chopped

2 cloves garlic, minced

2 tablespoons soy sauce

3 tablespoons teriyaki sauce

1 tablespoon neutral oil (canola or vegetable)

½ cup roasted and salted cashews

2 cups cooked white rice (for serving)

1. Heat oil in a large skillet or wok over medium-high heat.
2. Add chicken and cook for 5–7 minutes, stirring occasionally, until golden brown and cooked through. Remove from skillet and set aside.
3. In the same skillet, add peppers, onion, and garlic. Cook for 4–5 minutes until vegetables are softened.
4. Return chicken to the skillet and stir in soy sauce and teriyaki. Mix well until everything is coated in sauce.
5. Stir in cashews right before serving to keep them crunchy.
6. Serve hot over cooked white rice.

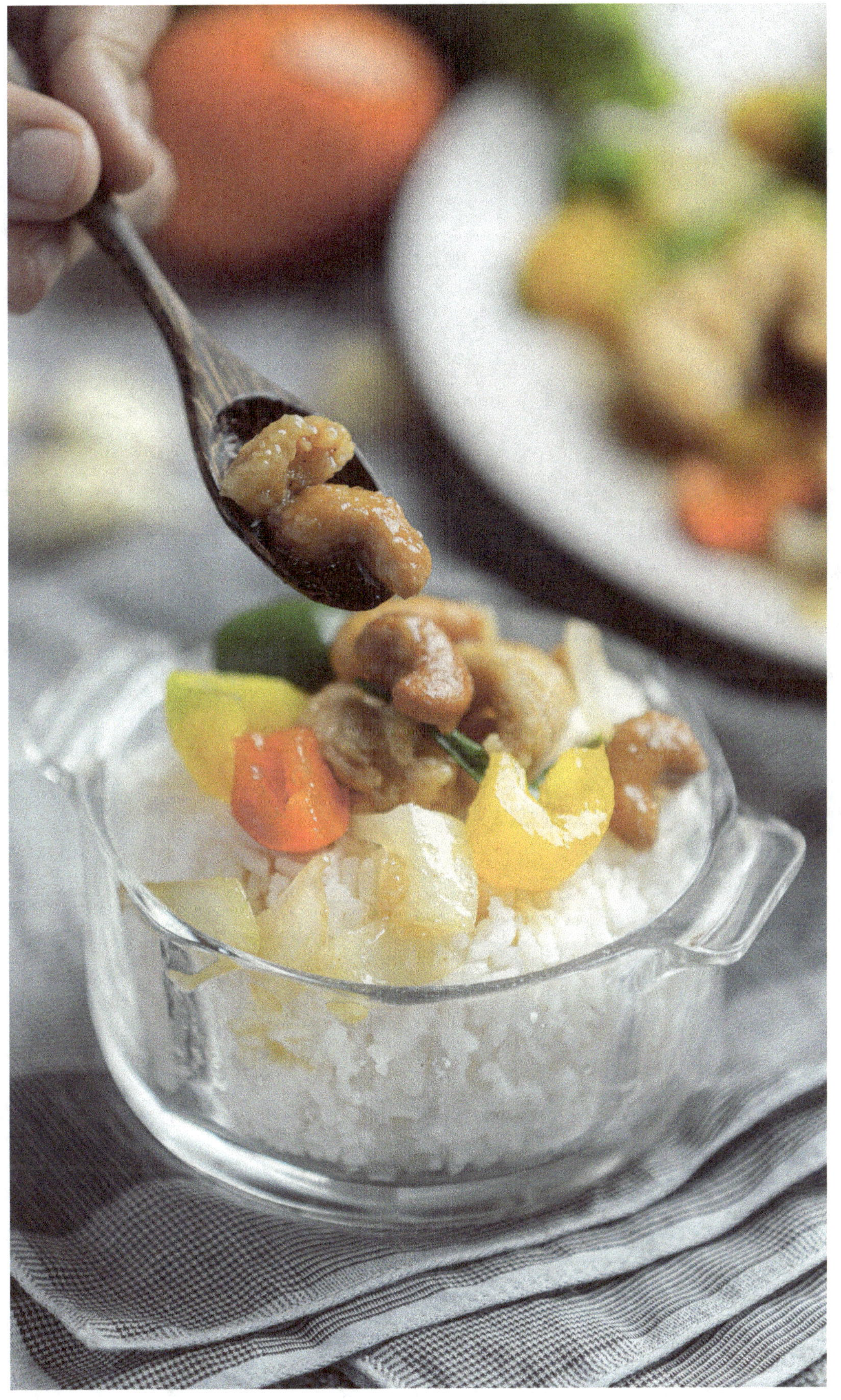

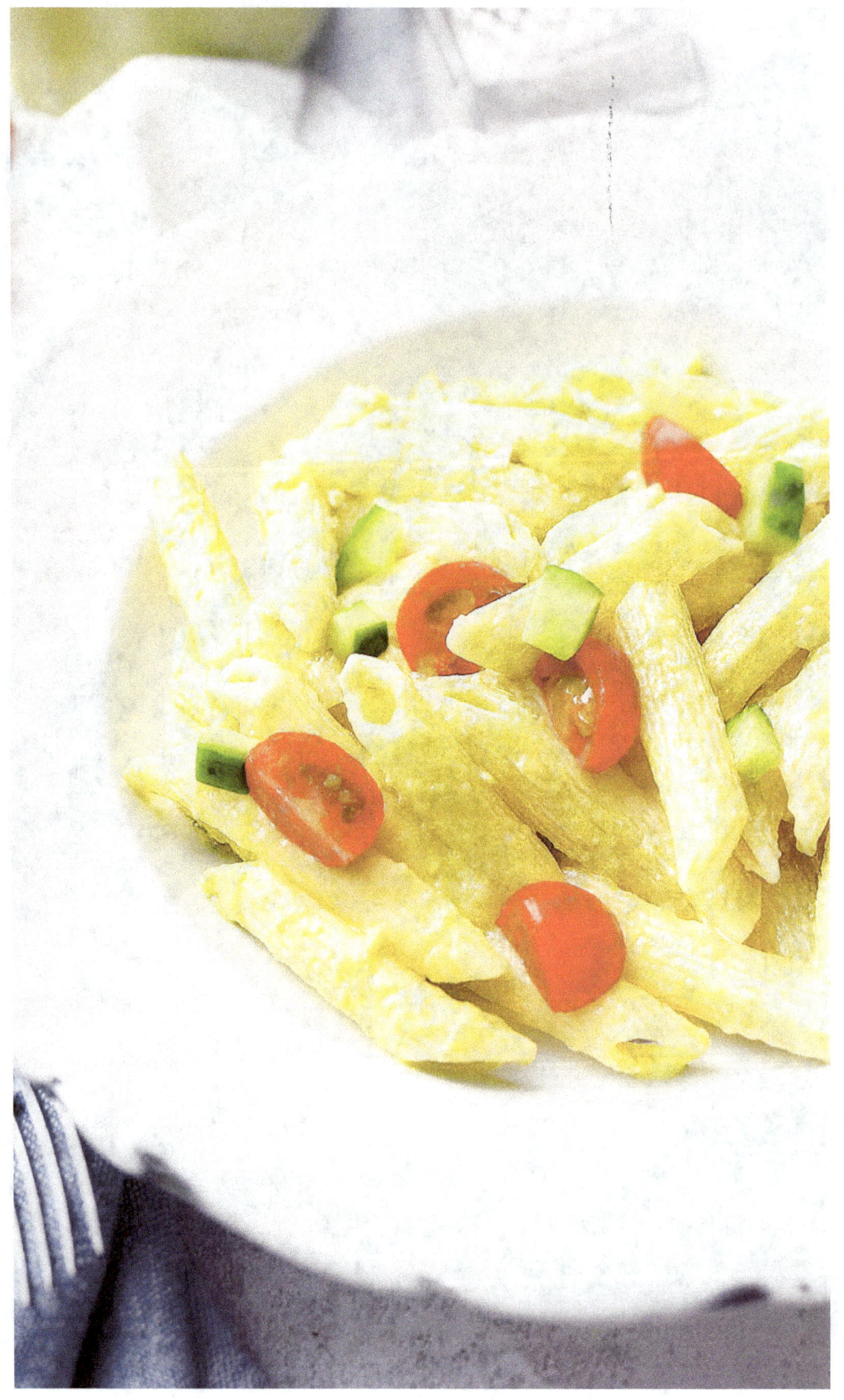

ROOM TEMPERATURE CREAMY PASTA SALAD

Spoon Rating: 🍴🍴🍴
Makes: 4–5 servings
Texture: Soft pasta, creamy dressing, crisp vegetables
Temperature: Room temperature
Prep Time: 15 minutes
Calories per serving: ~350–400
Sensory Notes: Creamy, mild flavors with crunch from veggies

Pasta salad is a flexible, sensory-friendly dish that works well when served at room temperature. No need to worry about eating it piping hot or ice cold. You can use your favorite pasta shape, and even premade filled pasta like tortellini works really well here for extra comfort and flavor. This recipe is mild and creamy, and you can easily adjust it with your preferred vegetables or seasonings.

12 oz pasta of choice (short pasta like rotini, penne, or premade tortellini)

½ cup mayonnaise or plain Greek yogurt (for lighter version)

1 tablespoon olive oil

1 tablespoon lemon juice or vinegar

½ teaspoon salt

¼ teaspoon pepper (optional)

1 small cucumber, diced (optional)

1 cup cherry tomatoes, halved (optional)

½ cup shredded cheese (mild cheddar or mozzarella)

1. Cook pasta according to package directions until tender. Drain and let cool to room temperature.
2. In a large bowl, whisk together mayonnaise (or yogurt), olive oil, lemon juice, salt, and pepper.
3. Add cucumber, cherry tomatoes (or preferred vegetables), and shredded cheese to the bowl.
4. Stir in cooled pasta until everything is evenly coated.
5. Taste and adjust seasoning as needed. Serve at room temperature.

CRISP CINNAMON SUGAR PITA CHIPS

Spoon Rating: 🍴🍴🍴
Makes: 3–4 servings
Texture: Crisp and crunchy
Temperature: Room temperature
Prep Time: 15 minutes
Calories per serving: ~180–220
Sensory Notes: Sweet, toasty, and crunchy with a warm cinnamon aroma

Pita chips are a fun, crunchy snack that give you the satisfaction of a crisp bite without being too heavy. These are lightly sweetened with cinnamon and sugar, and they pair perfectly with a sweet yogurt dip for balance. They also store well, so you can make them ahead and keep some ready for snack cravings.

3 white pita breads, cut into triangles

2 tablespoons melted butter or neutral oil

2 tablespoons granulated sugar

1 teaspoon cinnamon

1. Preheat oven to 375°F (190°C).
2. Place pita triangles on a baking sheet in a single layer.
3. Brush both sides of pita triangles with melted butter or oil.
4. Mix sugar and cinnamon in a small bowl, then sprinkle evenly over the pita pieces.
5. Bake for 8–10 minutes, flipping halfway through, until golden and crisp.
6. Let cool slightly before serving with your favorite sweet yogurt dip.

SILKY SWEET VANILLA YOGURT DIP

Spoon Rating: 🥄🥄
Makes: 2–3 servings
Texture: Silky and smooth
Temperature: Cold
Prep Time: 5 minutes
Calories per serving: ~120–150
Sensory Notes: Sweet, creamy, lightly floral vanilla with no tart aftertaste

This dip is creamy, smooth, and lightly sweet, making it a perfect companion for fruit, pita chips, or cookies. If the tartness of plain yogurt bothers you, the vanilla and honey balance it out and help neutralize those sharper flavors. It's quick to make and feels like a treat without much effort.

1 cup plain Greek yogurt (whole milk for extra creaminess)

2 tablespoons honey or maple syrup

1 teaspoon vanilla extract

1. In a medium bowl, combine yogurt, honey, and vanilla extract.
2. Stir until completely smooth and well blended.
3. Taste and adjust sweetness if needed by adding more honey or syrup.
4. Serve chilled with fruit, pita chips, or cookies.

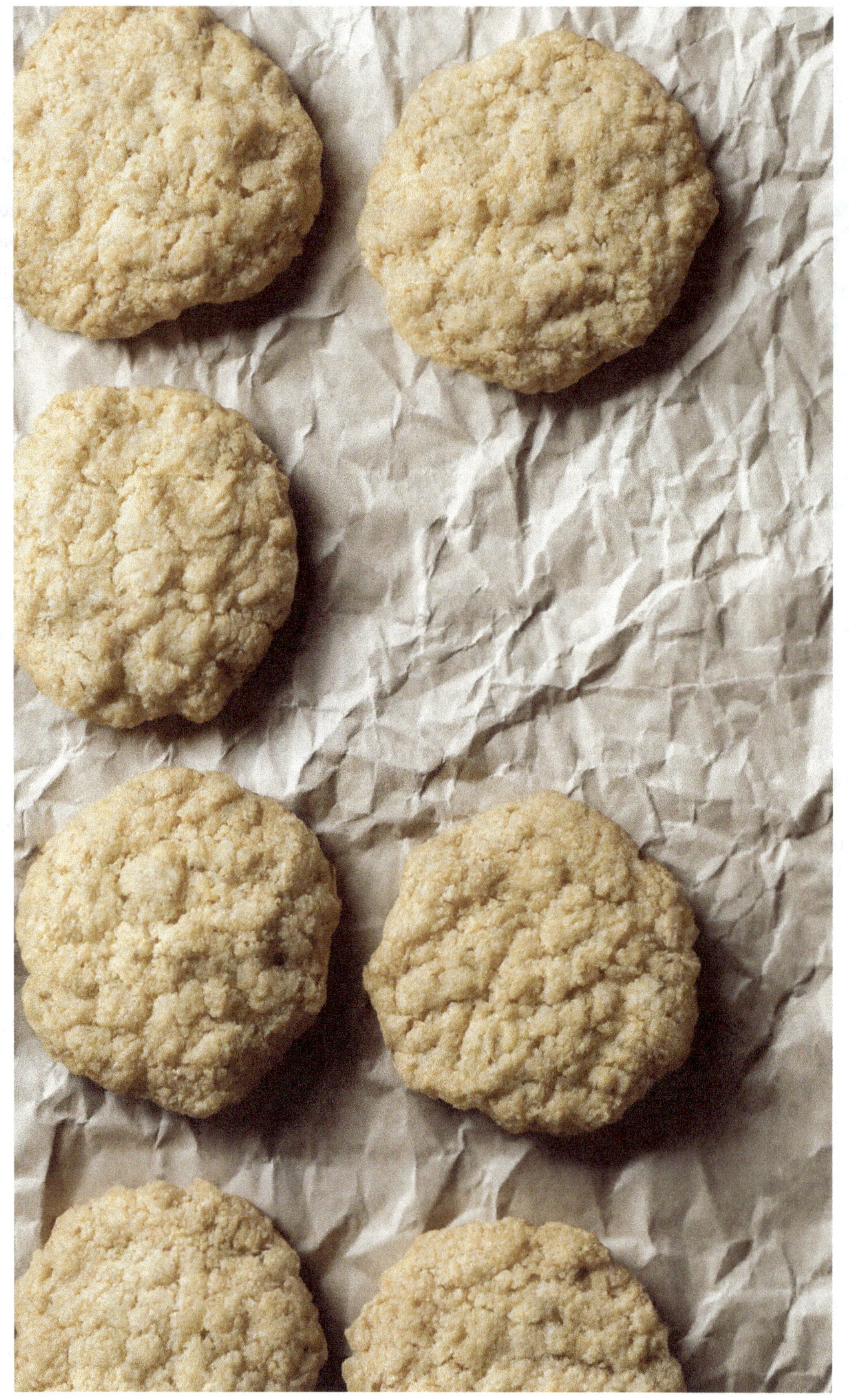

CHEWY OATMEAL COOKIES

Spoon Rating: 🍴🍴🍴
Makes: About 24 cookies
Texture: Soft and chewy inside, lightly crisp edges
Temperature: Warm
Prep Time: 15 minutes
Calories per serving: ~180 per cookie
Sensory Notes: Sweet, buttery, oat flavor with satisfying chew

These cookies are soft and chewy with just the right amount of sweetness. They're delicious on their own, but you can easily add raisins, chocolate chips, or even chopped nuts if you want a little extra texture or flavor. This base recipe is simple, reliable, and perfect for a comforting treat.

1 cup unsalted butter, softened

1 cup brown sugar, packed

½ cup white sugar

2 large eggs

2 teaspoons vanilla extract

1 ½ cups all-purpose flour

1 teaspoon baking soda

1 teaspoon cinnamon (optional)

½ teaspoon salt

3 cups rolled oats

1. Preheat oven to 350°F (175°C). Line a baking sheet with parchment paper.
2. In a large bowl, cream together butter, brown sugar, and white sugar until fluffy.
3. Beat in eggs and vanilla until smooth.
4. In another bowl, whisk flour, baking soda, cinnamon (if using), and salt.
5. Add dry ingredients to wet ingredients and mix until just combined.
6. Stir in oats until evenly distributed.
7. Scoop tablespoon-sized portions onto baking sheet, leaving space between cookies.
8. Bake for 10–12 minutes until edges are golden but centers still look soft.
9. Let cool on baking sheet for 5 minutes before transferring to a wire rack.

SUPER SMOOTH BANANA "ICE CREAM"

Spoon Rating: 🍴🍴🍴
Makes: 2 servings
Texture: Silky and creamy
Temperature: Cold
Prep Time: 5 minutes (plus freezing time)
Calories per serving: ~120–150
Sensory Notes: Naturally sweet, smooth, no added sugar, refreshing finish

This is the easiest way to make ice cream at home without needing a complicated machine. It uses frozen bananas blended until silky smooth. The natural sweetness of ripe bananas makes this a great base, and you can add flavors like vanilla, cocoa, or peanut butter if you want. The texture comes out like soft-serve, which makes it especially friendly for sensory-sensitive eaters.

3 ripe bananas, peeled, sliced, and frozen overnight

1 teaspoon vanilla extract (optional)

2–3 tablespoons milk or non-dairy milk, as needed for blending

1. Peel and slice ripe bananas and place them in a sealed bag or container. Freeze at least 6 hours or overnight.
2. Add frozen banana slices to a blender or food processor.
3. Blend, scraping down sides as needed, until mixture starts to look creamy.
4. Add vanilla and milk (a spoonful at a time) to help blend until completely smooth.
5. Serve immediately for soft-serve texture, or freeze for 1–2 hours for a firmer scoop.

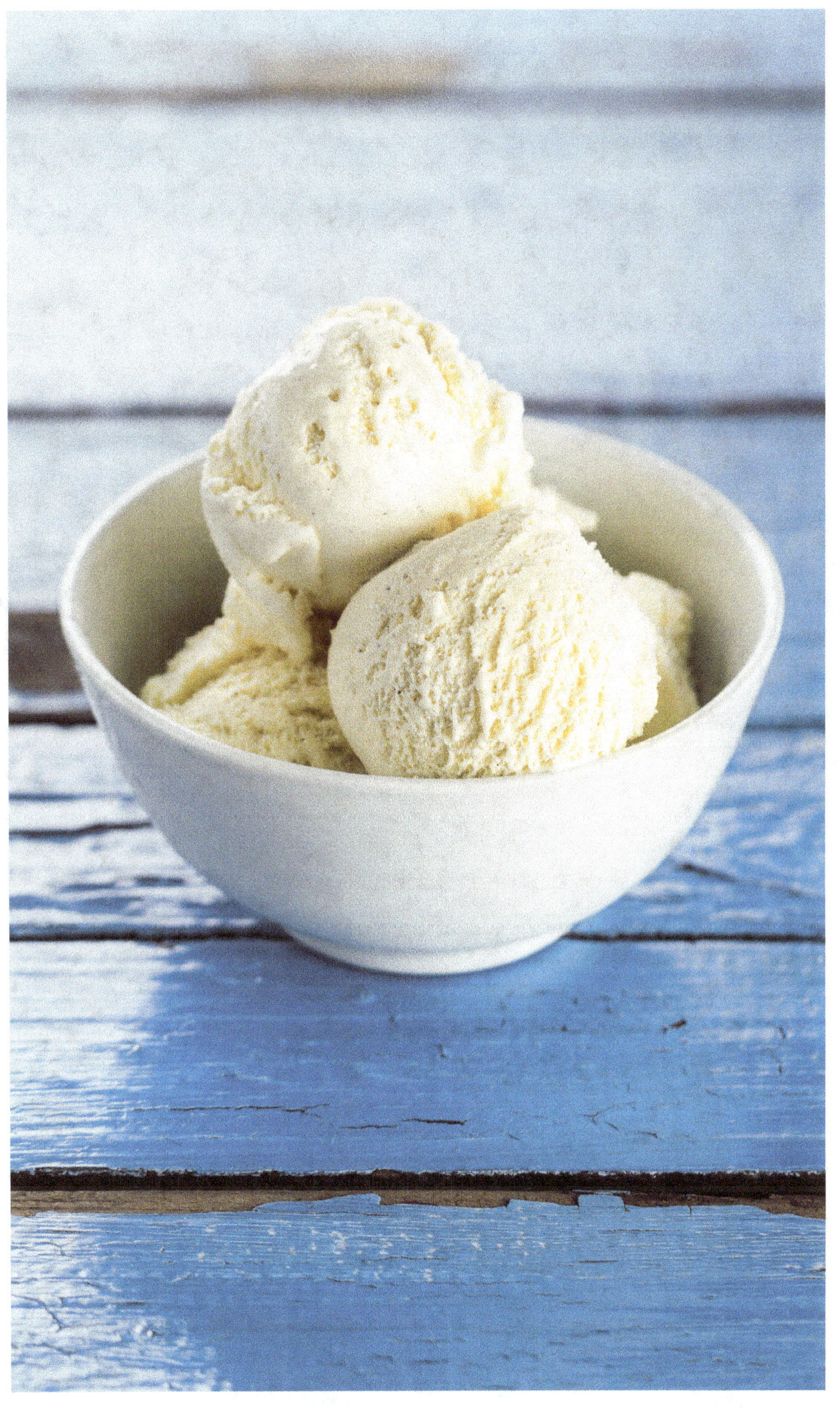

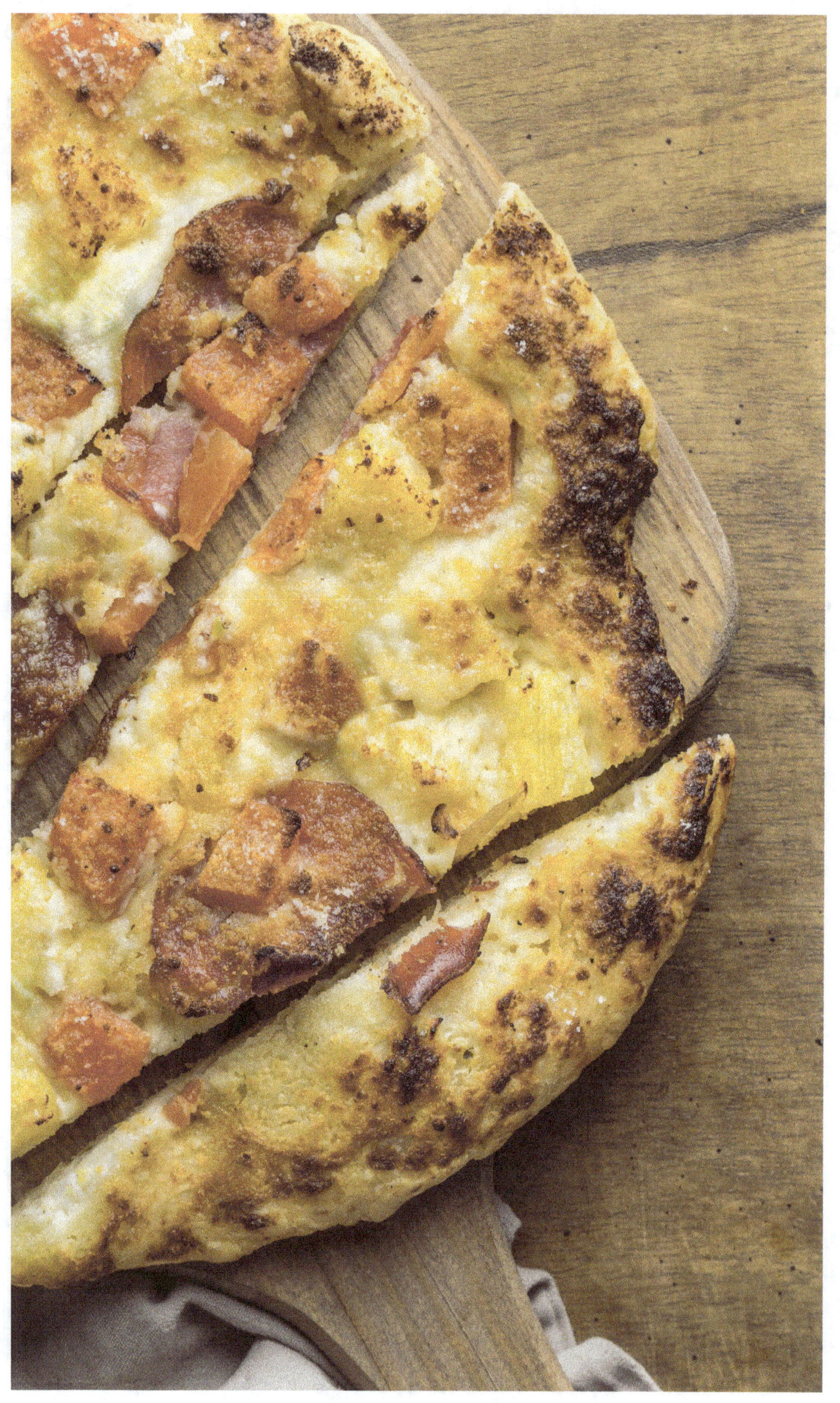

CHAPTER 8: SAFE FOOD TRANSFORMATIONS

Safe foods are the foundation of comfort and predictability. These are the go-to meals and snacks that feel reliable, consistent, and non-threatening. In this chapter, we'll look at ways to gently build on those safe foods so they can provide more nourishment without changing the familiar flavors or textures too much. The goal isn't to replace or take away what works, it's to layer in small, easy shifts that make your plate more supportive of your body's needs.

Think of it as making your safe foods "work harder" for you. By adding a little protein to a carb-based comfort food, blending in a mild vegetable to a favorite sauce, or topping something familiar with a sprinkle of healthy fats, you increase nutrition while keeping the core food recognizable. These transformations are subtle, not overwhelming. With time, small adjustments can create a big impact, giving you confidence and variety without disrupting the sense of safety you rely on at mealtime.

BUTTERNUT SQUASH MAC AND CHEESE

Spoon Rating: 🍴🍴🍴🍴
Makes: 3–4 servings
Texture: Creamy sauce with soft pasta
Temperature: Hot
Prep Time: 20 minutes
Calories per serving: ~350–400
Sensory Notes: Familiar cheesy flavor, smooth with no strong squash taste

Mac and cheese is a classic comfort food, and this version sneaks in a little extra nutrition without changing the taste too much. Butternut squash has a naturally mild, slightly sweet, neutral flavor that blends seamlessly with cheese sauce. When pureed, it creates a silky base that makes the sauce even creamier. Most grocery stores carry precut or even frozen butternut squash, which makes this recipe easier and less overwhelming than handling a whole squash.

8 oz elbow macaroni (or your favorite pasta shape)

2 cups cubed butternut squash (fresh precut or frozen)

1 cup milk (dairy or non-dairy)

1 ½ cups shredded mild cheddar cheese

2 tablespoons butter

1 teaspoon salt

½ teaspoon garlic powder (optional)

1. Bring a medium pot of water to a boil. Add the cubed squash and cook until tender, about 10–12 minutes. Remove squash with a slotted spoon and set aside.
2. In the same water, cook pasta according to package directions until tender. Drain and set aside.
3. Blend the cooked squash with milk until completely smooth.
4. Pour the squash puree into a saucepan over medium heat. Stir in butter, salt, garlic powder (if using), and shredded cheese. Mix until melted and creamy.
5. Add cooked pasta to the sauce and stir until well coated. Serve warm.

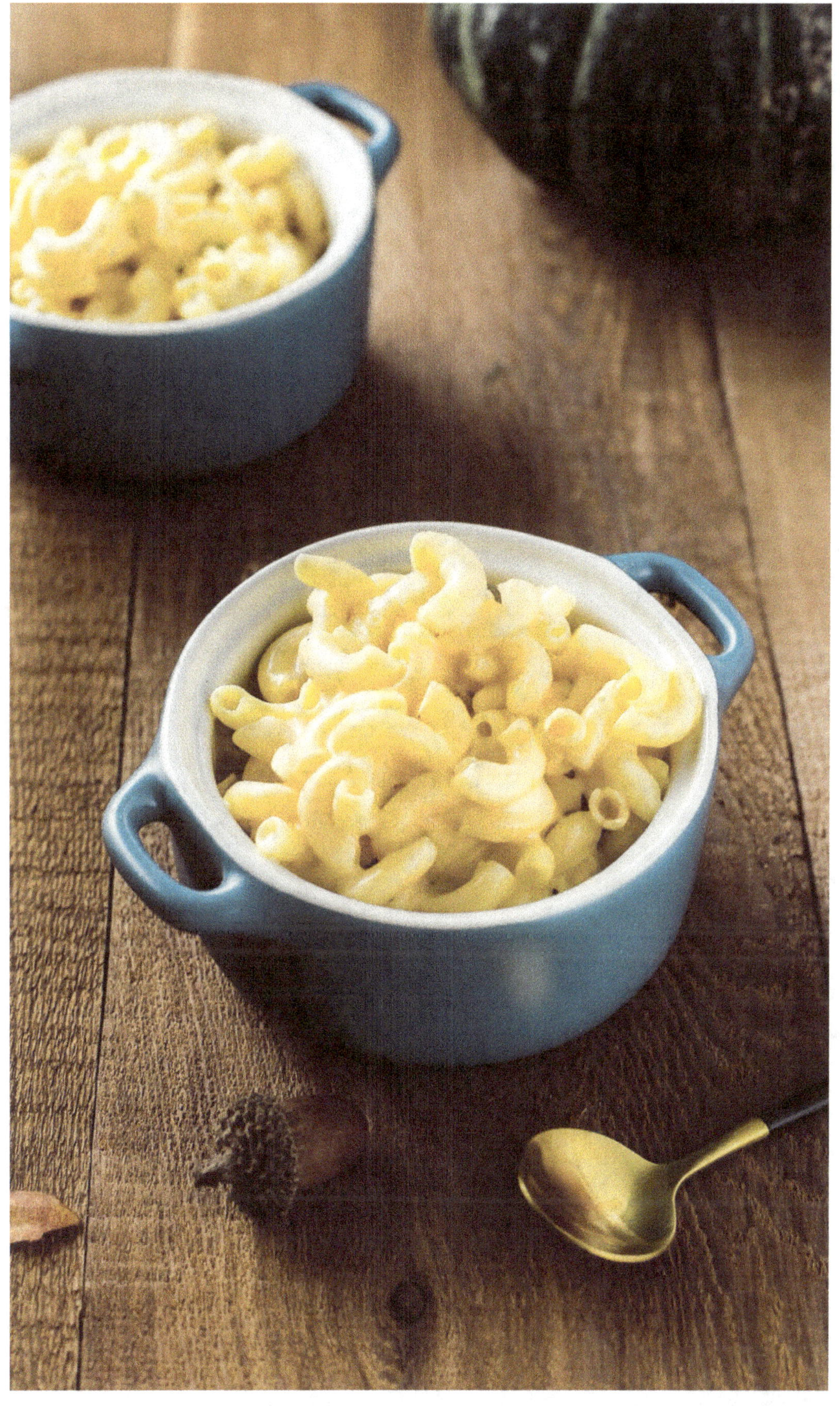

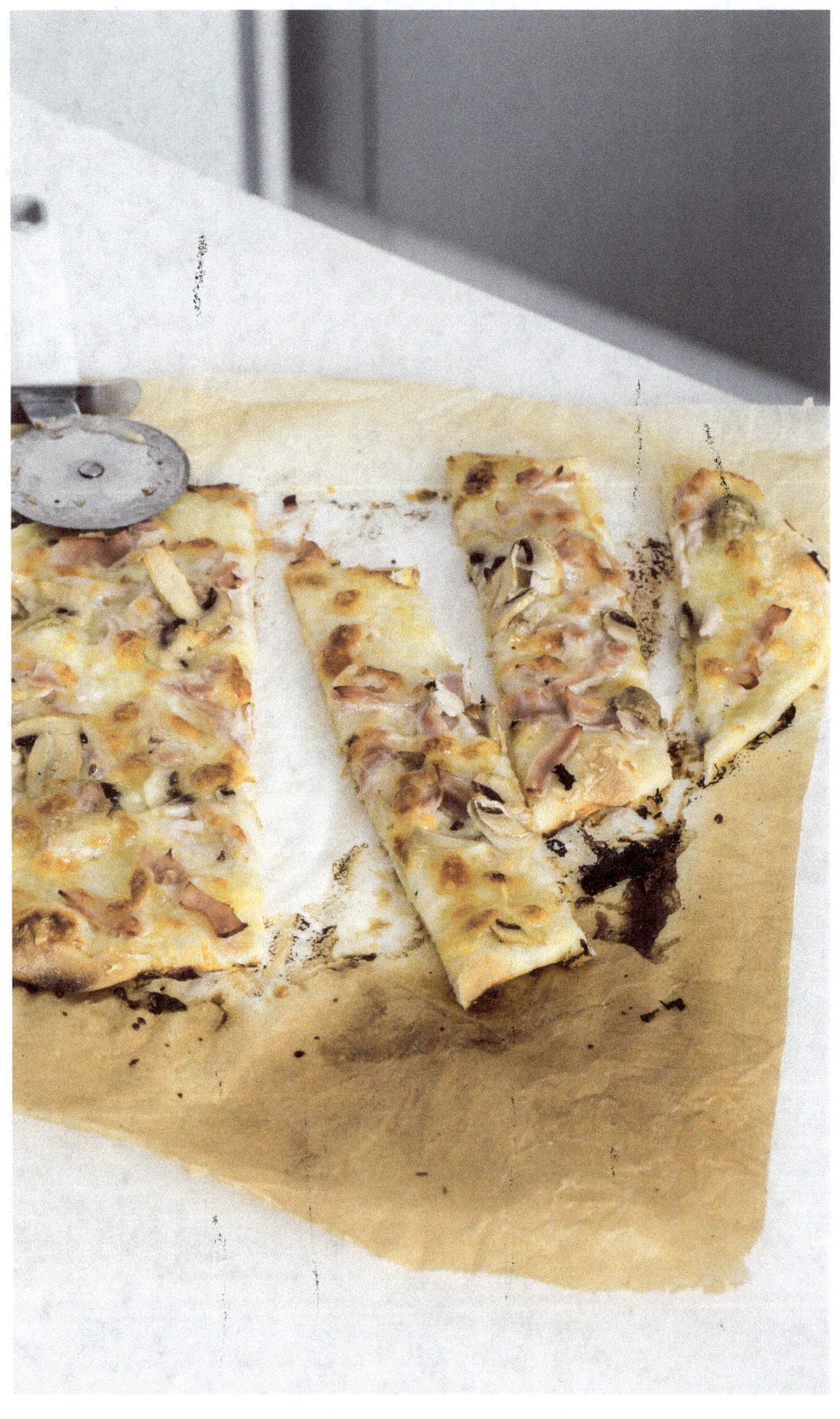

PIZZA WITH CAULIFLOWER CRUST

Spoon Rating:
Makes: 2–3 servings
Texture: Crispy edges, soft but firm center
Temperature: Hot
Prep Time: 20 minutes
Calories per serving: ~300–350 (without extra toppings)
Sensory Notes: Familiar pizza flavors, mild cauliflower base

Pizza is one of the most reliable comfort foods, but for some neurodivergent eaters, bread can feel too heavy. A cauliflower crust lightens things up while still delivering a familiar, cheesy pizza flavor. Cauliflower has a neutral taste, and when baked into a crust, it holds toppings well without being overwhelming. Most grocery stores carry pre-riced cauliflower (fresh or frozen), which saves you from having to prep a whole head of cauliflower.

3 cups riced cauliflower (fresh or frozen, thawed and squeezed dry)

1 cup shredded mozzarella cheese

¼ cup grated Parmesan cheese

1 egg, beaten

½ teaspoon salt

½ teaspoon garlic powder (optional)

½ cup pizza sauce (store-bought or homemade)

1 cup shredded mozzarella (for topping)

Optional toppings: pepperoni, sliced veggies, or just keep it plain cheese

1. Preheat oven to 425°F (220°C). Line a baking sheet or pizza pan with parchment paper.
2. If using frozen riced cauliflower, thaw and squeeze out as much moisture as possible with a clean towel. This is important for a crisp crust.
3. In a large bowl, combine cauliflower, mozzarella, Parmesan, egg, salt, and garlic powder. Mix until well combined.
4. Press the mixture onto the parchment-lined pan, shaping into a thin, even circle or rectangle.
5. Bake for 20–25 minutes, until golden and firm.
6. Remove from oven, spread pizza sauce on top, then sprinkle with mozzarella and any toppings you like.
7. Return to the oven and bake for another 8–10 minutes, until cheese is melted and bubbly.
8. Slice and serve warm.

PLAIN PASTA WITH HIDDEN VEGGIE SAUCE

Spoon Rating: 🥄🥄🥄🥄
Makes: 2–3 servings
Texture: Soft pasta, smooth sauce
Temperature: Hot
Prep Time: 20 minutes
Calories per serving: ~350–400
Sensory Notes: Familiar pasta base, mild veggie flavors hidden in smooth sauce

Sometimes the best way to introduce more nutrition is by blending it right into familiar flavors. This recipe uses your favorite plain pasta paired with a smooth, hidden veggie sauce that feels and tastes like a classic tomato sauce but has extra nutrients. Carrots, zucchini, or even spinach can disappear into the mix once blended, so you get the comfort of pasta with a boost of vegetables without noticing. Using jarred marinara as the base keeps prep simple and executive-function-friendly.

8 oz pasta of choice (any shape, your favorite works)

1 cup jarred marinara sauce

1 small carrot, peeled and chopped

½ zucchini, chopped

1 handful baby spinach (optional)

1 tablespoon olive oil

½ teaspoon salt (adjust to taste)

¼ teaspoon garlic powder (optional)

2 tablespoons grated Parmesan cheese (optional, for topping)

1. Bring a pot of salted water to a boil and cook pasta according to package directions. Drain and set aside.
2. In a small pan, heat olive oil over medium heat. Add carrot and zucchini, sautéing for 5–7 minutes until softened. Add spinach for the last minute if using.
3. Transfer cooked vegetables to a blender or food processor. Add marinara sauce, salt, and garlic powder. Blend until completely smooth.
4. Pour sauce back into the pan and heat gently for 3–4 minutes, stirring.
5. Toss pasta with sauce until well coated.
6. Serve warm, topped with Parmesan if desired.

VEGGIE-PACKED MEATBALLS

Spoon Rating: ⚲⚲
Makes: 3–4 servings
Texture: Soft inside, lightly crisp outside
Temperature: Hot
Prep Time: 25 minutes
Calories per serving: ~300–350
Sensory Notes: Familiar savory flavor, vegetables blended in for hidden nutrition, tender bite

Meatballs are a familiar, comforting food, and they can also be a great way to sneak in extra nutrition without changing the flavor too much. By finely grating or blending vegetables into the mix, you get all the moisture and nutrients while keeping the taste mild and familiar. Using ground sirloin makes these meatballs less greasy than regular beef, but you can also use ground chicken or turkey for a lighter option. Serve them with pasta and sauce, in a sandwich, or even on their own as a protein-packed snack.

1 lb ground sirloin, chicken, or turkey

1 small carrot, finely grated

½ zucchini, finely grated and squeezed to remove excess water

¼ small onion, finely grated or blended

1 egg, beaten

½ cup plain breadcrumbs

½ teaspoon salt

¼ teaspoon pepper (optional, mild flavor)

½ teaspoon garlic powder (optional)

1 cup jarred marinara sauce (optional, for serving)

1. In a large bowl, combine ground meat, grated carrot, grated zucchini, onion, egg, breadcrumbs, salt, and seasonings. Mix gently until just combined.

2. Use a spoon or small scoop to form even-sized meatballs, about 1 ½ inches in diameter.

3. For oven: Preheat to 400°F (200°C). Line a baking sheet with parchment paper. Place meatballs on the baking sheet and bake for 18–20 minutes, until browned and cooked through (internal temp 165°F for poultry, 160°F for beef).

4. For air fryer: Preheat to 375°F (190°C). Arrange meatballs in a single layer, spray lightly with cooking spray, and cook for 12–14 minutes, shaking halfway through, until browned and cooked through.

5. Optionally, warm marinara sauce in a saucepan and toss meatballs in sauce before serving.

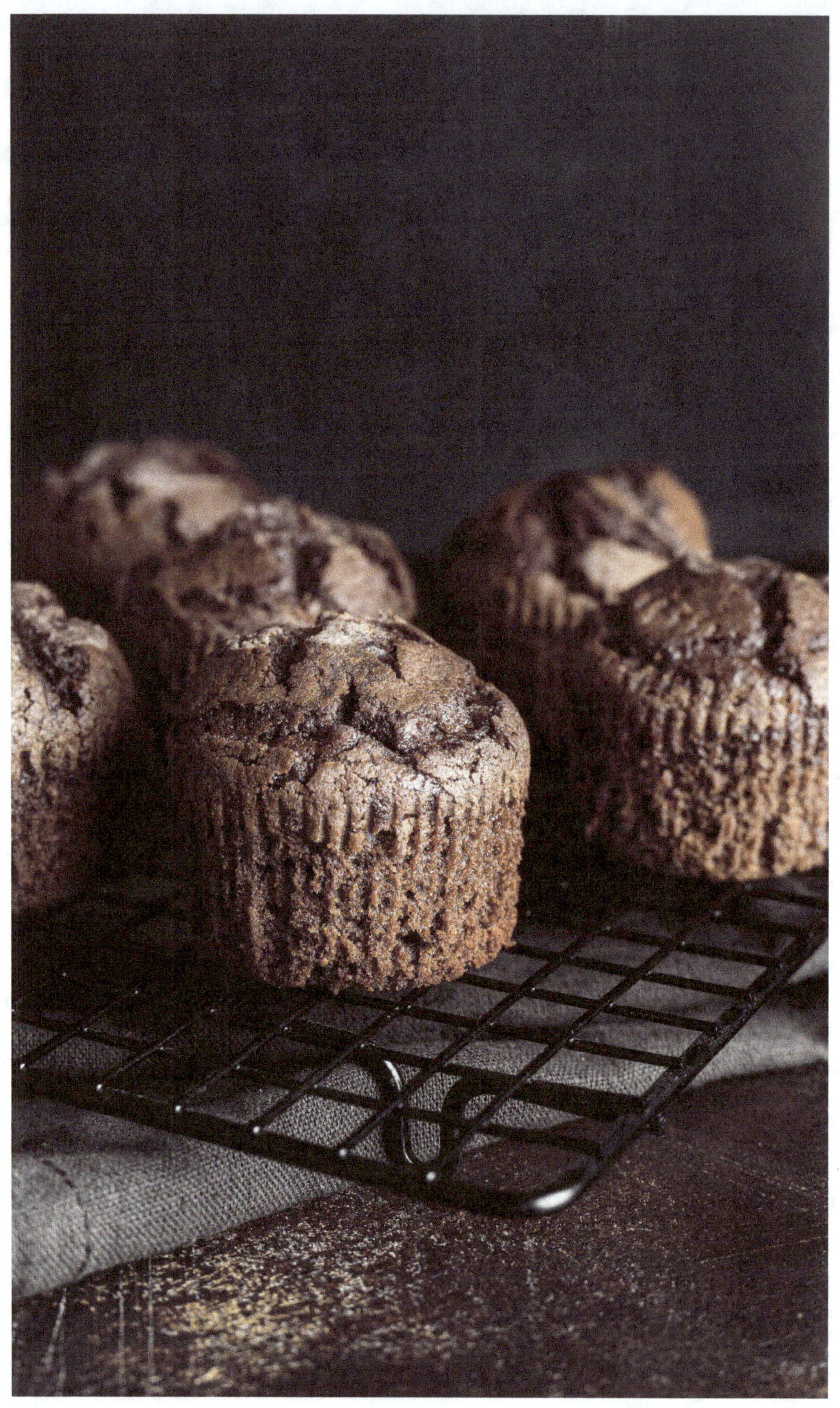

ZUCCHINI CHOCOLATE MUFFINS

Spoon Rating: 🥄🥄🥄🥄
Makes: 10–12 muffins
Texture: Soft and moist
Temperature: Warm or room temperature
Prep Time: 15 minutes
Calories per serving: ~180–200
Sensory Notes: Chocolate flavor, zucchini blends in invisibly, familiar muffin bite

These muffins are a perfect example of a safe food transformation. They look and taste like a classic chocolate treat, but they sneak in extra nutrition thanks to shredded zucchini. The zucchini adds moisture and softness without changing the flavor, making them approachable even for selective eaters. They're also a great make-ahead option for quick snacks or breakfast on the go.

1 cup finely grated zucchini (about 1 small zucchini, squeezed of extra liquid)

1 cup all-purpose flour

½ cup cocoa powder

½ teaspoon baking powder

½ teaspoon baking soda

¼ teaspoon salt

2 eggs

½ cup sugar

¼ cup neutral oil (or melted butter)

¼ cup milk (dairy or non-dairy)

1 teaspoon vanilla extract

½ cup chocolate chips (optional, for extra sweetness)

1. Preheat oven to 350°F (175°C). Line a muffin tin with paper liners or lightly grease.
2. In a medium bowl, whisk together flour, cocoa powder, baking powder, baking soda, and salt.
3. In a separate large bowl, whisk together eggs, sugar, oil, milk, and vanilla until smooth.
4. Stir grated zucchini into the wet mixture.
5. Gradually fold the dry ingredients into the wet mixture until just combined. Do not overmix.
6. If using, fold in chocolate chips.
7. Divide batter evenly into muffin cups, filling about ¾ full.
8. Bake for 18–20 minutes, until a toothpick inserted in the center comes out clean. Let cool slightly before serving.

SWEET POTATO PANCAKES

Spoon Rating: 🍴🍴🍴
Makes: 6–8 pancakes
Texture: Soft, fluffy, with a gentle chew
Temperature: Hot
Prep Time: 20 minutes
Calories per serving: ~150–170
Sensory Notes: Mildly sweet, cozy flavor, familiar pancake texture with a subtle twist

Sweet potatoes are naturally sweet, soft, and mild, which makes them a great ingredient for transforming classic pancakes into something a little more nourishing. Using mashed sweet potato gives these pancakes extra fluffiness and a subtle flavor that blends right in without being overwhelming. You can use canned sweet potato purée to skip the prep, or roast and mash your own ahead of time.

1 cup all-purpose flour

1 teaspoon baking powder

½ teaspoon cinnamon (optional, mild flavor)

¼ teaspoon salt

1 egg

½ cup mashed sweet potato (canned or homemade)

¾ cup milk (dairy or non-dairy)

2 tablespoons neutral oil or melted butter

1 tablespoon sugar or honey

2 tablespoons neutral oil or coconut oil for frying

1. In a medium bowl, whisk together flour, baking powder, cinnamon (if using), and salt.
2. In a large bowl, whisk together egg, mashed sweet potato, milk, oil, and sugar until smooth.
3. Gradually fold the dry ingredients into the wet mixture until just combined. Do not overmix.
4. Heat a nonstick skillet over medium-low heat and add a small amount of oil or coconut oil.
5. Pour about ¼ cup batter per pancake into the skillet. Cook for 2–3 minutes, until bubbles form on the surface, then flip and cook another 2–3 minutes until golden and set.
6. Serve warm with butter, syrup, or your favorite topping.

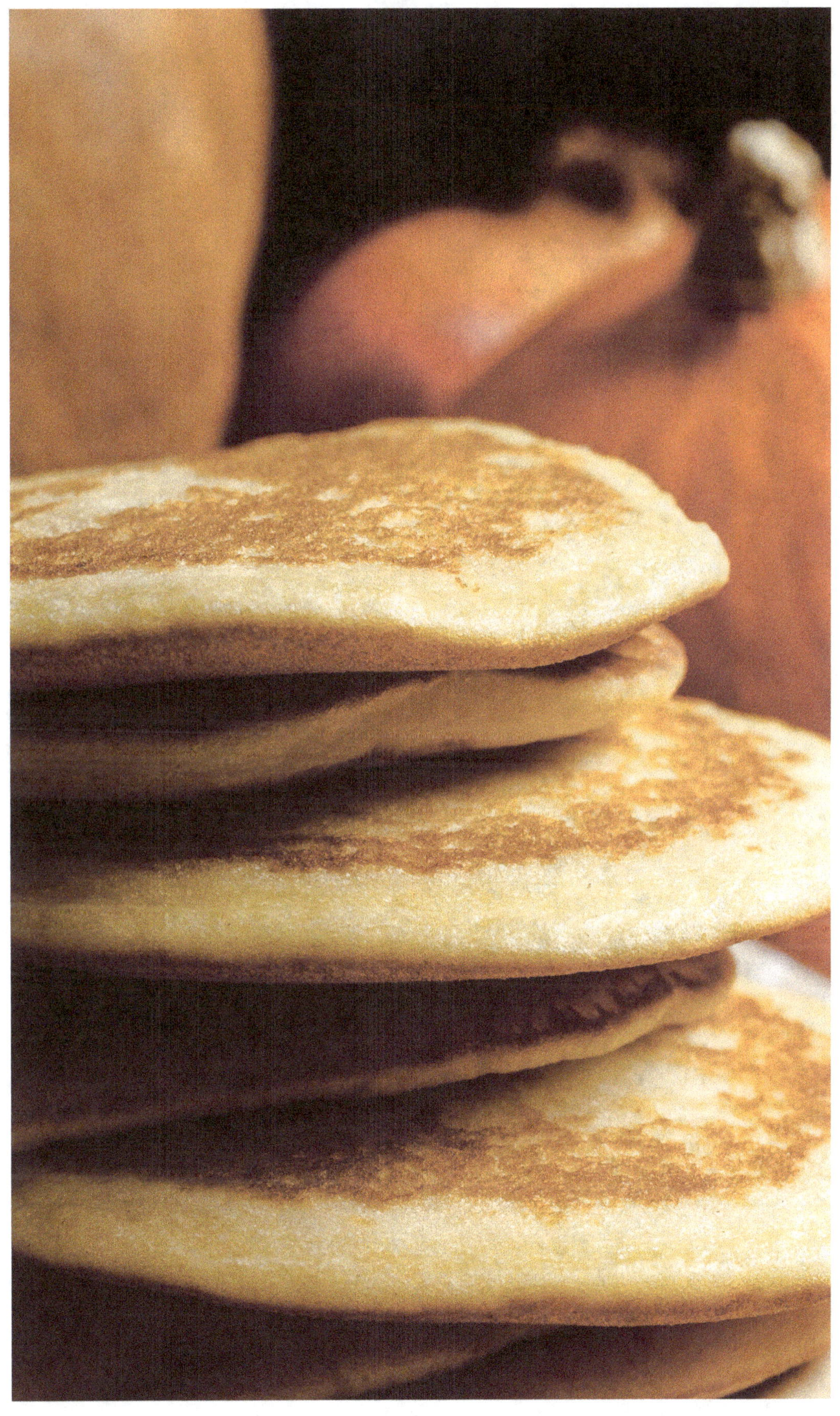

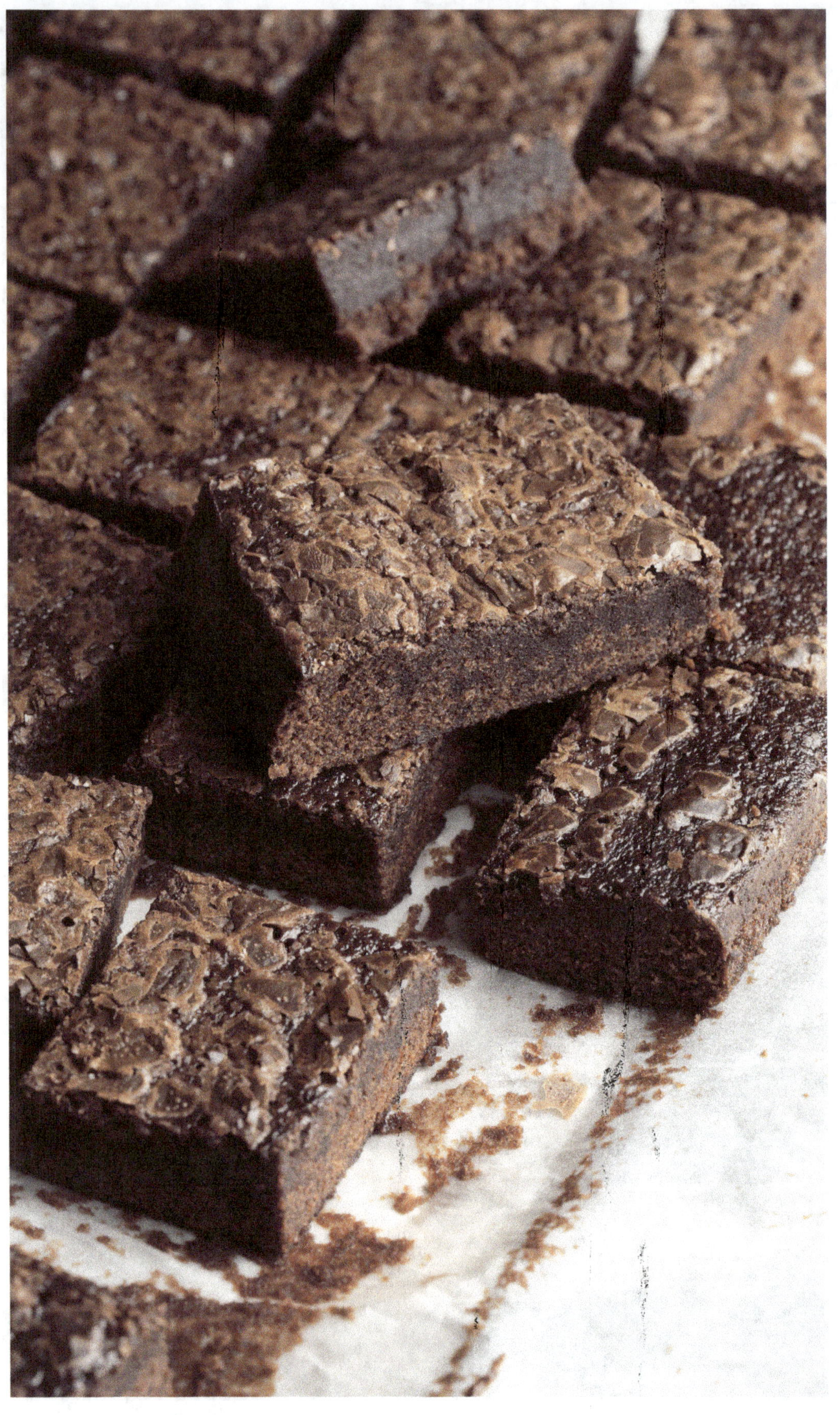

HIDDEN VEGGIE BROWNIES

Spoon Rating: 🍴🍴🍴
Makes: 9–12 brownies
Texture: Fudgy and soft, chewy
Temperature: Warm or room temperature
Prep Time: 15 minutes
Calories per serving: ~180–200
Sensory Notes: Rich chocolate flavor, smooth and moist, no obvious veggie taste

Brownies are a comfort classic, and this version sneaks in a little extra nutrition without changing the familiar taste and texture. Pureed vegetables like zucchini or sweet potato add moisture and richness, making the brownies extra soft and fudgy while still tasting like dessert. People won't notice the veggies are there. It's an easy win for getting more variety into your safe foods.

1 cup all-purpose flour

½ cup cocoa powder

1 teaspoon baking powder

¼ teaspoon salt

½ cup mashed sweet potato or zucchini puree (well-drained if using zucchini)

½ cup sugar

½ cup neutral oil or melted butter

2 eggs

1 teaspoon vanilla extract

½ cup chocolate chips (optional, for extra sweetness)

1. Preheat oven to 350°F (175°C). Grease or line an 8x8-inch baking dish with parchment paper.
2. In a medium bowl, whisk together flour, cocoa powder, baking powder, and salt.
3. In a large bowl, mix the sweet potato or zucchini puree with sugar, oil, eggs, and vanilla until smooth.
4. Add dry ingredients into the wet mixture and stir until just combined. Fold in chocolate chips if using.
5. Pour batter into prepared pan and spread evenly.
6. Bake for 22–25 minutes, until the center is set but still slightly soft for a fudgy texture. Do not overbake.
7. Let cool before slicing into squares.

SECRETLY NUTRITIOUS COOKIES

Spoon Rating: 🥄🥄🥄
Makes: 12–14 cookies
Texture: Soft and chewy
Temperature: Room temperature or warm
Prep Time: 20 minutes
Calories per serving: ~130–150
Sensory Notes: Mild sweetness, warm spice, moist bite with no strong veggie flavor

These cookies taste like a soft, cozy treat, but they're boosted with pumpkin or sweet potato puree for extra nutrition and natural sweetness. The puree also keeps the cookies moist and chewy, so they stay soft for days. You can enjoy them as-is or mix in a handful of chocolate chips for extra indulgence.

1 cup all-purpose flour

½ teaspoon baking soda

½ teaspoon cinnamon

¼ teaspoon salt

½ cup of canned pumpkin or sweet potato puree (well-drained if watery)

½ cup sugar (brown sugar works well for extra softness)

¼ cup neutral oil or melted butter

1 egg

1 teaspoon vanilla extract

½ cup chocolate chips or chopped nuts (optional)

1. Preheat oven to 350°F (175°C). Line a baking sheet with parchment paper.
2. In a medium bowl, whisk together flour, baking soda, cinnamon, and salt.
3. In a large bowl, mix the pumpkin or sweet potato puree with sugar, oil, egg, and vanilla until smooth.
4. Add dry ingredients to wet mixture and stir until just combined. Fold in chocolate chips or nuts if using.
5. Scoop dough into tablespoon-sized portions and place on baking sheet about 2 inches apart.
6. Bake for 10–12 minutes, until cookies are set but still soft in the center.
7. Let cool on the pan for 5 minutes before transferring to a wire rack.

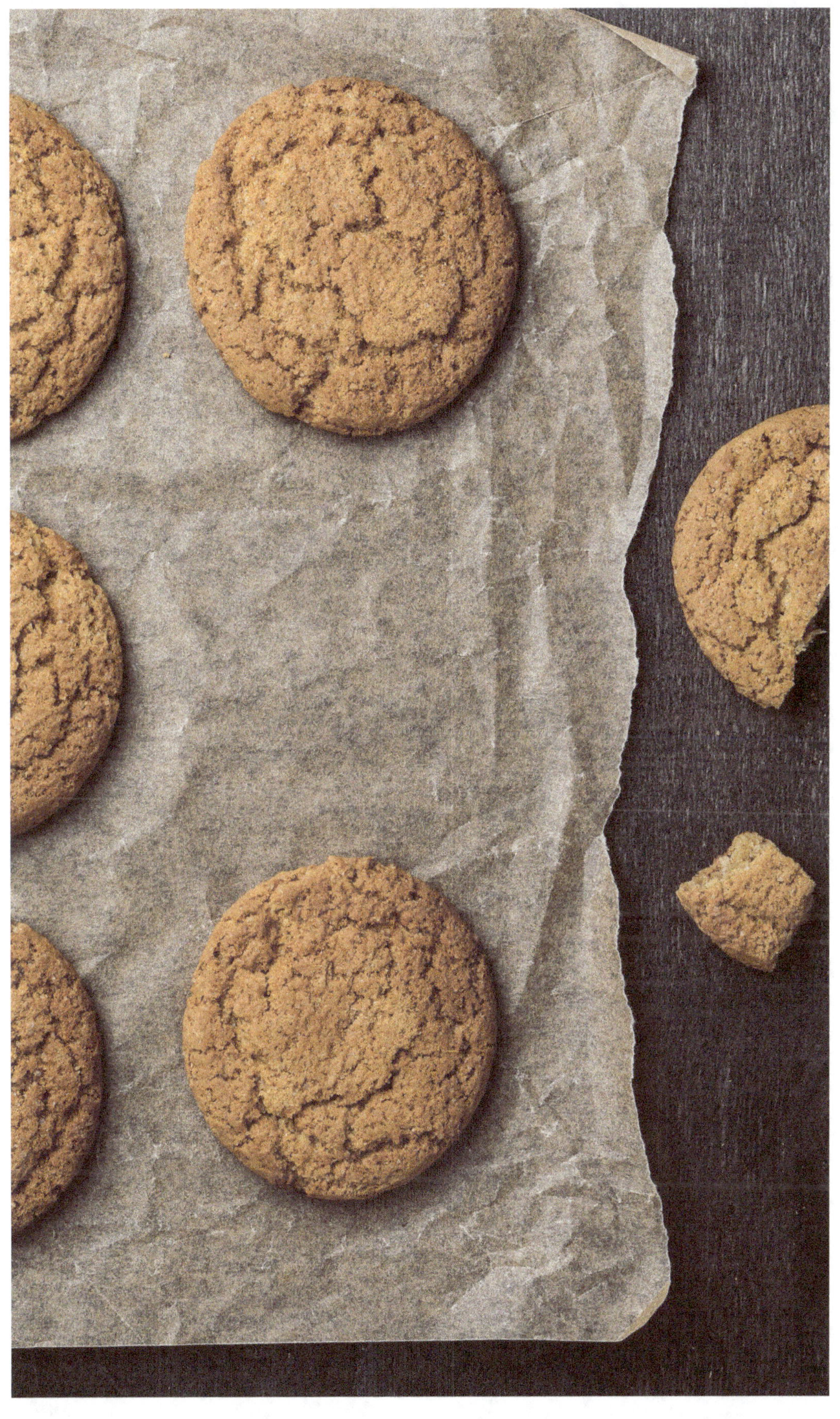

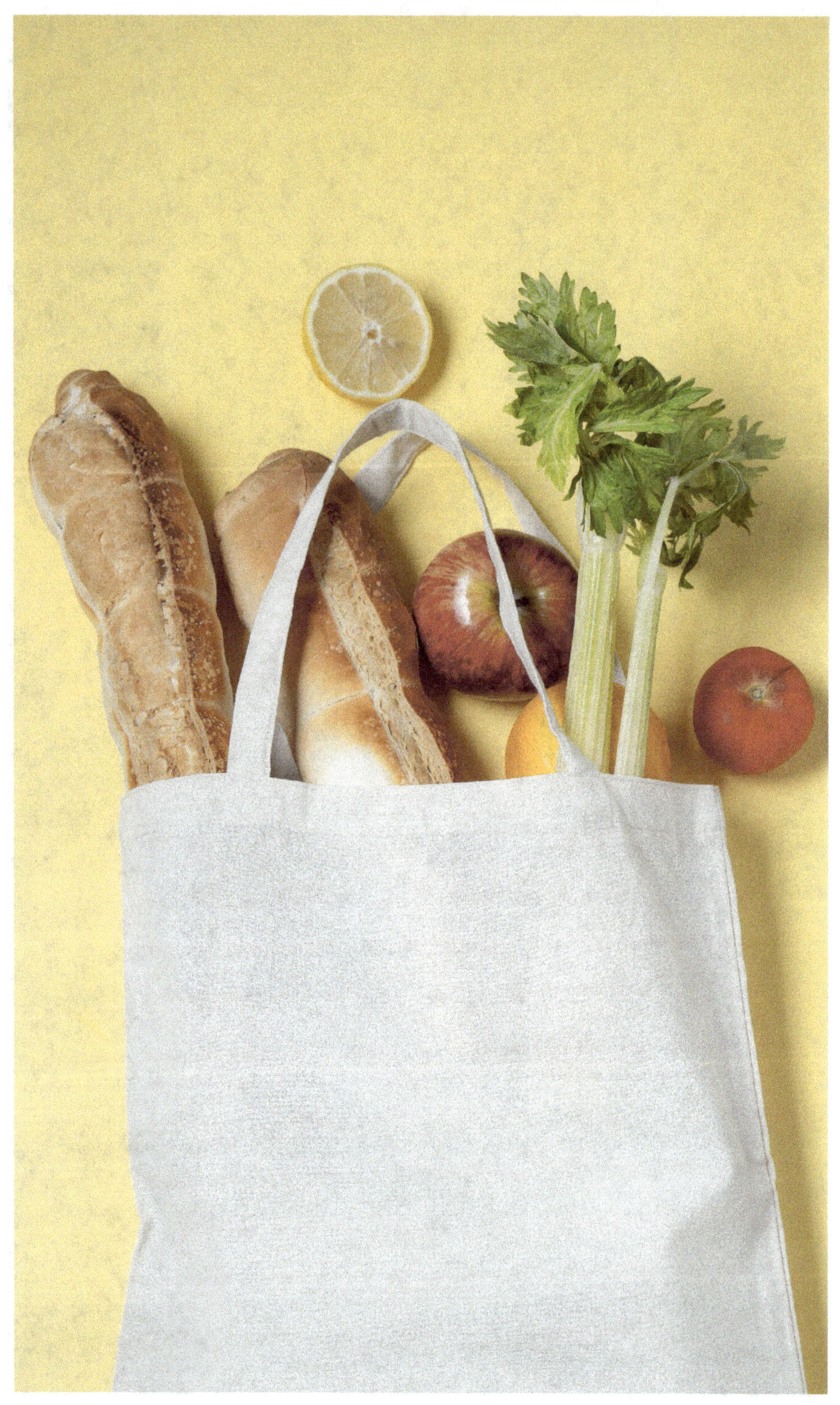

CHAPTER 9: EXECUTIVE FUNCTION FRIENDLY

Cooking takes more than just following a recipe. It requires planning, remembering steps, switching between tasks, and cleaning as you go. For many neurodivergent people, these "invisible" demands are harder than the cooking itself. That's why this chapter focuses on meals that cut down the number of decisions you need to make. These recipes either cook once and feed you more than once, let you prep ahead for the week, or come together with simple assembly so there's very little to manage in the moment.

The goal here isn't gourmet cooking, it's creating reliable, low-stress meals you can actually make when your energy is running low. Think casseroles that stretch into leftovers, sheet pan meals that handle themselves in the oven, or build-it-yourself plates with easy store-bought foods. By setting yourself up with food that works harder for you, you'll spend less time thinking about what to eat and more time actually eating.

EASY SHEET PAN CHEESY NACHOS

Spoon Rating: 🍴🍴🍴
Makes: 4 servings
Texture: Crispy chips, gooey cheese
Temperature: Hot
Prep Time: 5 minutes
Calories per serving: ~400–500 (depending on toppings)
Sensory Notes: Crunchy, cheesy, customizable

Nachos are one of the simplest comfort meals to assemble when energy is low. The base recipe just needs chips and cheese, but you can layer on whatever toppings work best for you. Using a sheet pan keeps everything evenly melted and easy to grab.

1 large bag tortilla chips

2 cups shredded cheese (cheddar, Monterey Jack, or a Mexican blend)

Optional Add-Ons:

Cooked ground beef or ground sirloin

Cooked shredded chicken

Black beans or pinto beans (drained and rinsed)

Salsa or pico de gallo

Jalapeño slices

Sour cream

Guacamole

Avocado slices

Cilantro

1. Preheat oven to 375°F (190°C).
2. Spread tortilla chips in a single layer on a large sheet pan.
3. Sprinkle shredded cheese evenly over the chips.
4. Add any toppings you'd like to bake (such as beans, shredded chicken, or ground beef).
5. Bake for 8–10 minutes, or until cheese is fully melted and chips are warm.
6. Remove from oven and add fresh toppings like salsa, sour cream, or guacamole before serving.

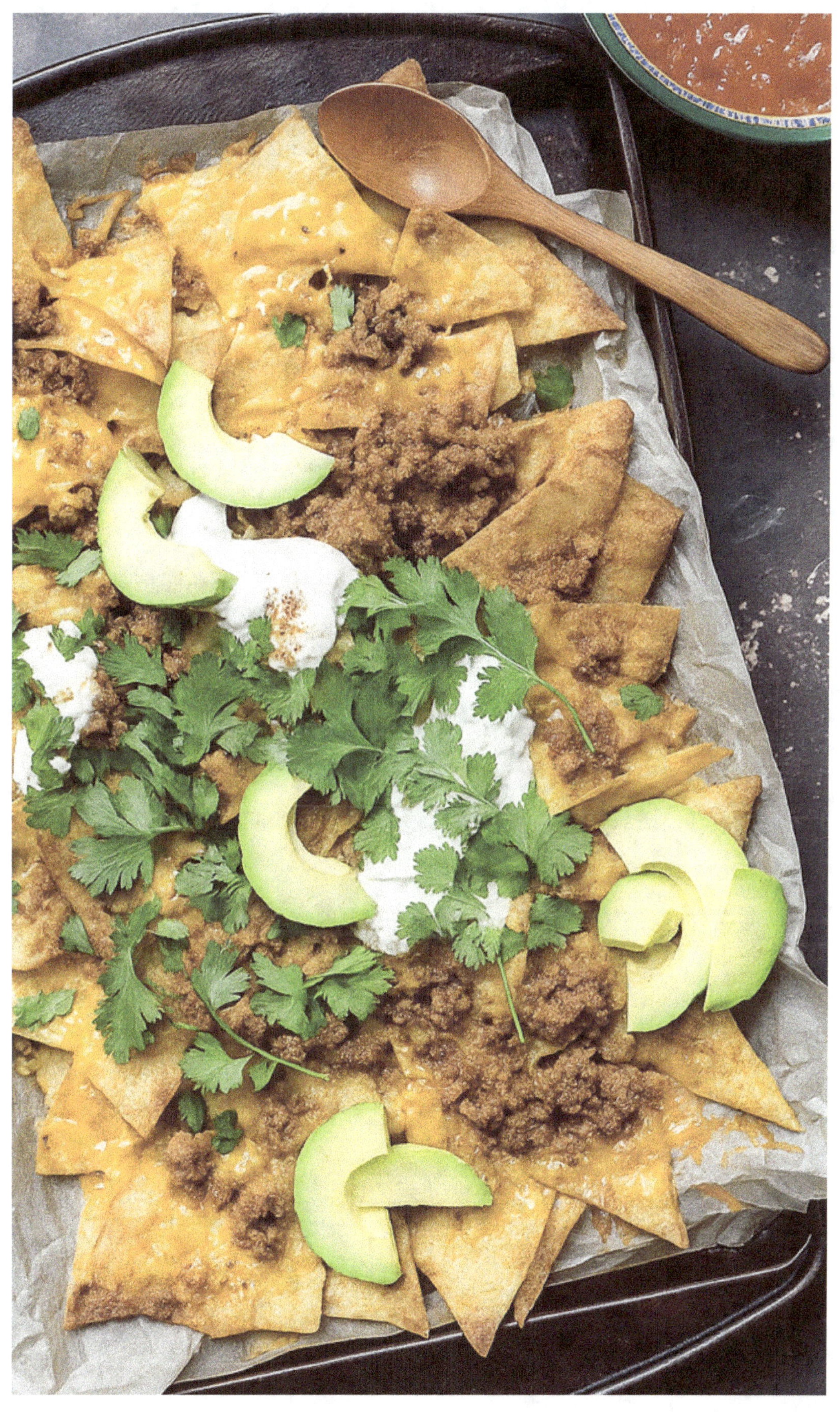

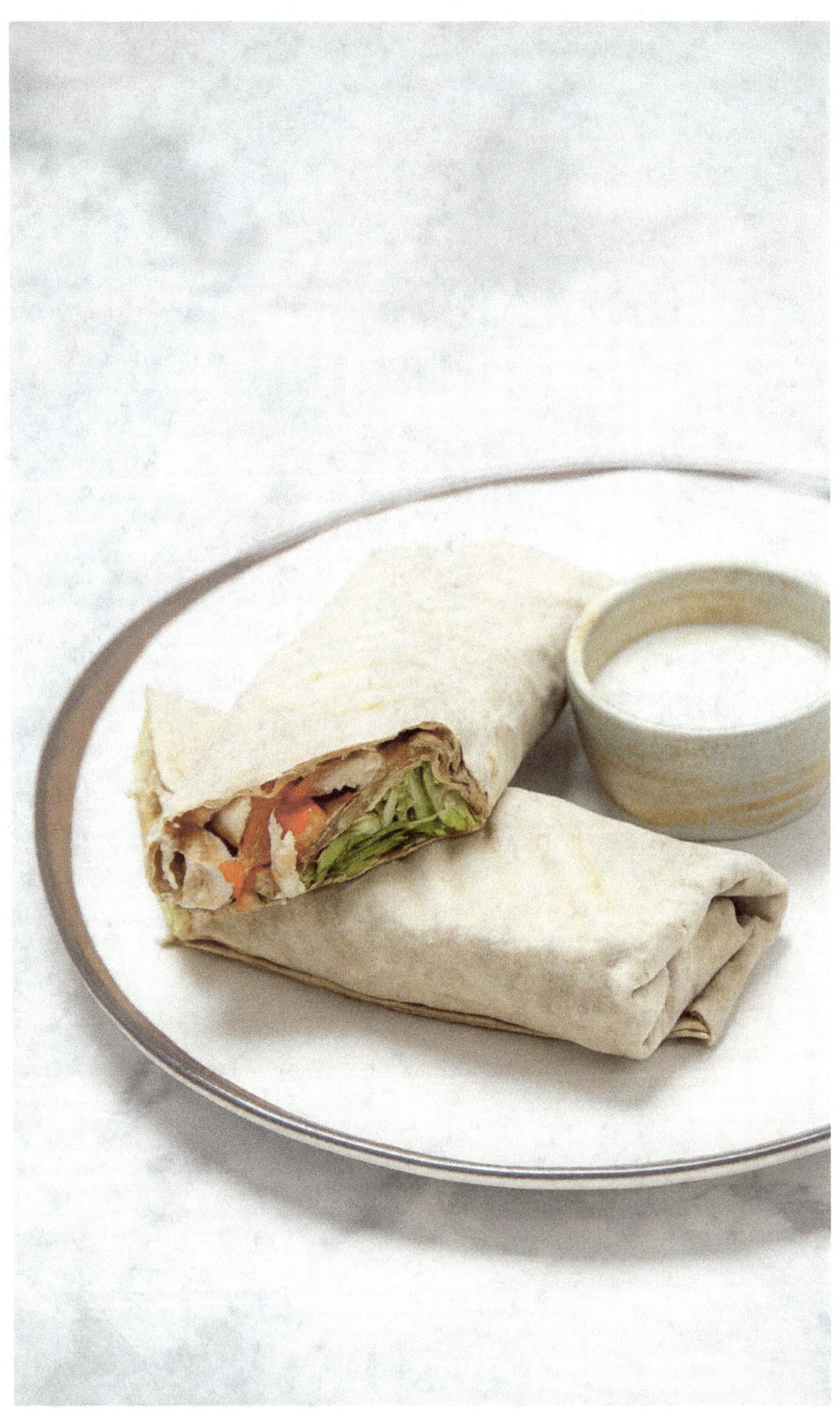

WRAP AND ROLL LUNCH

Spoon Rating: 🥄🥄🥄
Makes: 1 wrap
Texture: Soft tortilla, crisp lettuce, melty or cool cheese
Temperature: Cold or warm
Prep Time: 5–10 minutes
Calories per serving: ~300–350
Sensory Notes: Fresh, mild, customizable

Wraps are a quick, flexible meal that can be eaten cold or grilled for a warm, melty version. The base here uses turkey, cheese, tomato, and lettuce, but you can swap ingredients easily to match what feels best. If you prefer a toasted wrap, use a skillet or panini press to warm it until the cheese melts.

1 large flour tortilla (10–12 inch)

3–4 slices deli turkey

1 slice cheese (American, cheddar, or Swiss)

2 slices tomato (optional)

1–2 leaves lettuce (optional)

1 teaspoon mayonnaise or mustard (optional)

1. Lay the tortilla flat on a plate or cutting board.
2. Spread mayonnaise or mustard lightly over the tortilla, if using.
3. Layer turkey, cheese, tomato, and lettuce in the center.
4. Fold in the sides, then roll up tightly into a wrap.
5. For a warm version: place the wrap seam side down in a skillet over medium heat. Cook 2–3 minutes per side until lightly golden and cheese melts.
6. Slice in half and serve.

SHEET PAN CHICKEN AND VEGETABLES

Spoon Rating: ⫯⫯⫯
Makes: 3–4 servings
Texture: Juicy chicken, tender-crisp vegetables
Temperature: Hot
Prep Time: 10 minutes
Calories per serving: ~350–400
Sensory Notes: Mild flavor, colorful, balanced

This recipe is perfect for a balanced, one-pan dinner with minimal cleanup. Chicken breast provides lean protein, while roasted vegetables bring color and variety to the plate. If handling raw chicken feels overwhelming, you can wear disposable gloves or ask the butcher to precut the chicken into cubes so prep feels easier. Use whatever vegetables you prefer in place of what is listed here.

1 lb chicken breast, cut into bite-sized pieces

2 cups broccoli florets (or use pre-cut bagged broccoli)

1 red bell pepper, sliced into strips

1 zucchini, sliced into half-moons

2 tablespoons olive oil

1 teaspoon salt

½ teaspoon pepper (optional, mild flavor)

½ teaspoon garlic powder (optional)

1. Preheat oven to 400°F (200°C). Line a sheet pan with parchment paper or foil.
2. Place chicken pieces and vegetables on the sheet pan.
3. Drizzle with olive oil and sprinkle with salt, pepper, and garlic powder if using. Toss gently to coat everything evenly.
4. Spread into a single layer so pieces aren't crowded.
5. Roast for 20–25 minutes, stirring halfway through, until chicken reaches 165°F (75°C) and vegetables are tender-crisp.
6. Serve warm as-is, or over rice or pasta for a complete meal.

ONE-POT CREAMY PASTA

Spoon Rating: 🍴🍴🍴
Makes: 4 servings
Texture: Velvety, creamy sauce with tender pasta
Temperature: Hot
Prep Time: 5 minutes
Calories per serving: ~450–500
Sensory Notes: Mild, rich, comforting

This creamy pasta comes together in a single pot, making it an easy comfort meal with minimal cleanup. The cream cheese melts into the sauce to create a velvety texture that clings to the pasta beautifully. Everything cooks together, so you don't need to juggle multiple pans or steps. You can add premade shredded chicken or your favorite sauteed vegetable to add more flavors.

12 oz pasta (penne, rotini, or shells work well)

1 tablespoon olive oil or butter

3 cloves garlic, minced (or 1 teaspoon garlic powder for milder flavor)

3 cups low-sodium chicken or vegetable broth

1 cup milk

4 oz cream cheese, cut into cubes

1 cup shredded mozzarella or cheddar cheese

½ cup grated parmesan cheese (optional)

½ teaspoon salt

½ teaspoon pepper (optional)

1 teaspoon Italian seasoning (optional, mild flavor)

1. In a large pot, heat olive oil or butter over medium heat. Add garlic and cook for 1 minute until fragrant.
2. Add uncooked pasta, broth, and milk directly to the pot. Stir well and bring to a gentle boil.
3. Reduce heat to medium-low and cook, stirring occasionally, until pasta is tender and most liquid is absorbed (about 12–15 minutes).
4. Add cream cheese cubes and stir until fully melted into the sauce.
5. Stir in shredded cheese (and parmesan if using) until everything is creamy and smooth.
6. Taste and adjust with salt, pepper, or extra seasonings if desired. Serve hot.

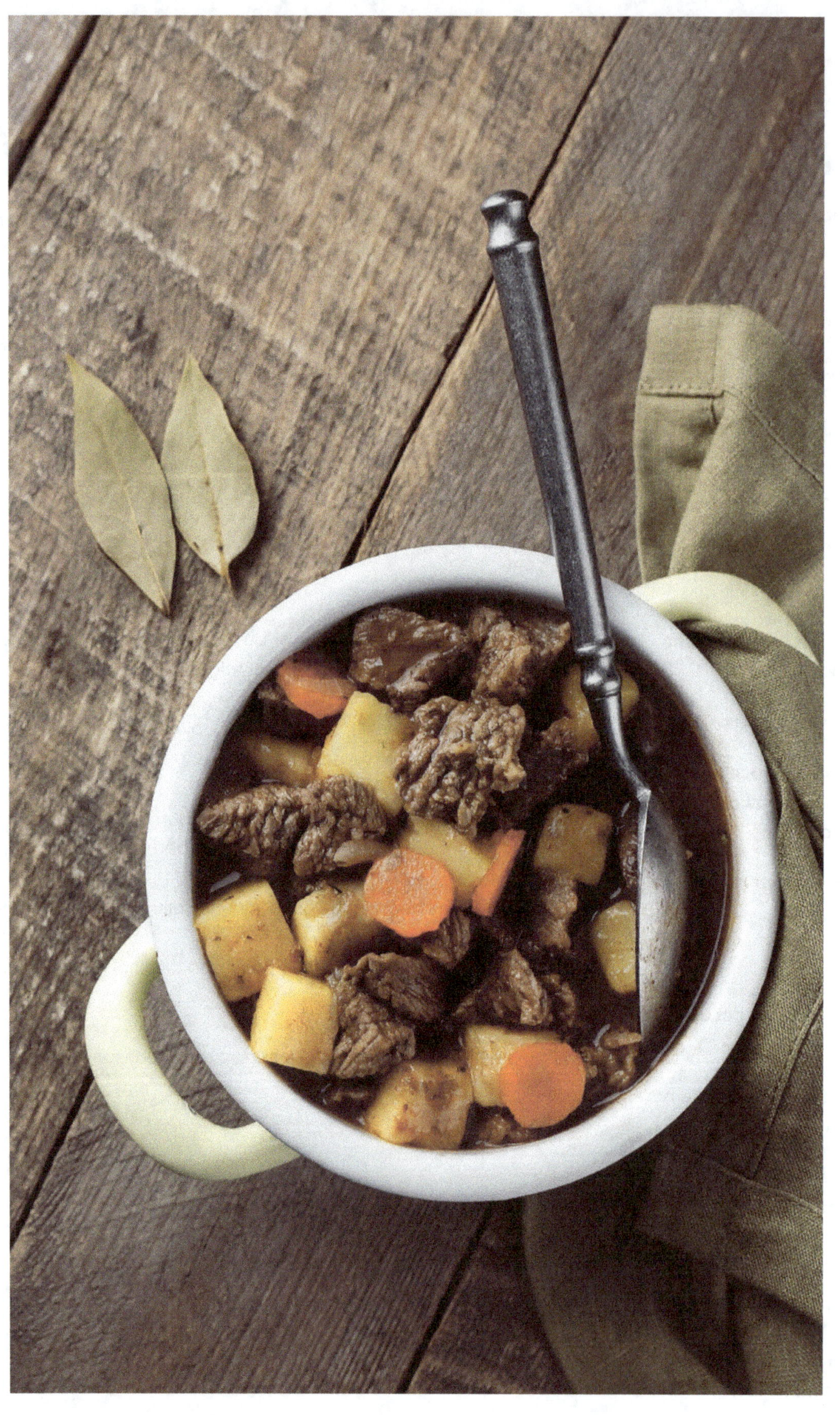

THROW-AND-GO SLOW COOKER BEEF STEW

Spoon Rating: 🍴🍴
Makes: 4 servings
Texture: Tender beef, soft vegetables, hearty broth
Temperature: Hot
Prep Time: 5 minutes
Calories per serving: ~400–450
Sensory Notes: Rich, savory flavor, deeply comforting

This hearty beef stew comes together with almost no effort, just drop everything in the slow cooker and walk away. The beef turns tender and the vegetables soak up rich, savory flavors, giving you a satisfying, homey meal with almost no hands-on cooking. It's the kind of dish that feels slow-cooked and comforting, but really only takes a few minutes of prep.

1 ½ lbs beef stew meat, cut into cubes (or buy pre-cut)

2 cups carrots, sliced

2 cups diced potatoes (or use bagged pre-chopped potatoes)

1 small onion, chopped (optional, or use pre-chopped)

2 cups beef broth (low-sodium if preferred)

1 teaspoon salt

½ teaspoon pepper (optional)

1 teaspoon dried thyme or Italian seasoning (optional)

1. Place beef, carrots, potatoes, and onion directly into the slow cooker.
2. Pour beef broth over everything.
3. Sprinkle with salt, pepper, and thyme/Italian seasoning.
4. Stir lightly or leave as is.
5. Cover and cook on low for 7–8 hours or high for 4–5 hours, until beef is tender and vegetables are soft.
6. Taste and adjust seasoning if needed before serving.

SNACK PLATE DINNER

Spoon Rating: 🍴
Makes: 1 serving
Texture: Mix of crunchy, soft, and creamy
Temperature: Room
Prep Time: 5 minutes
Calories per serving: ~400–600 (depending on items chosen)
Sensory Notes: Variety of flavors and textures

Sometimes dinner doesn't have to be cooked at all. A snack plate, or a small charcuterie board, is a fun and low-stress way to make a meal feel special. You can mix and match simple store-bought items like cheese, fruit, crackers, and a few sweet treats for a balanced plate that feels satisfying without much effort. This is a perfect option when energy is low or cooking feels overwhelming.

A few slices of cheese (cheddar, mozzarella, gouda, or your favorite)

Crackers or baguette slices

Fresh fruit (grapes, apple slices, or berries work well)

Raw veggies (baby carrots, cucumber slices, or bell peppers)

Small handful of nuts (optional)

A couple of cookies or a piece of chocolate for something sweet

Optional extras: deli turkey or ham, hummus, or store-bought dips

1. Arrange cheese, crackers or bread, fruit, and veggies on a plate or small board.
2. Add nuts and something sweet to round out the flavors.
3. If using deli meats or dips, place them in small piles or bowls.
4. Enjoy as a mix-and-match dinner plate.

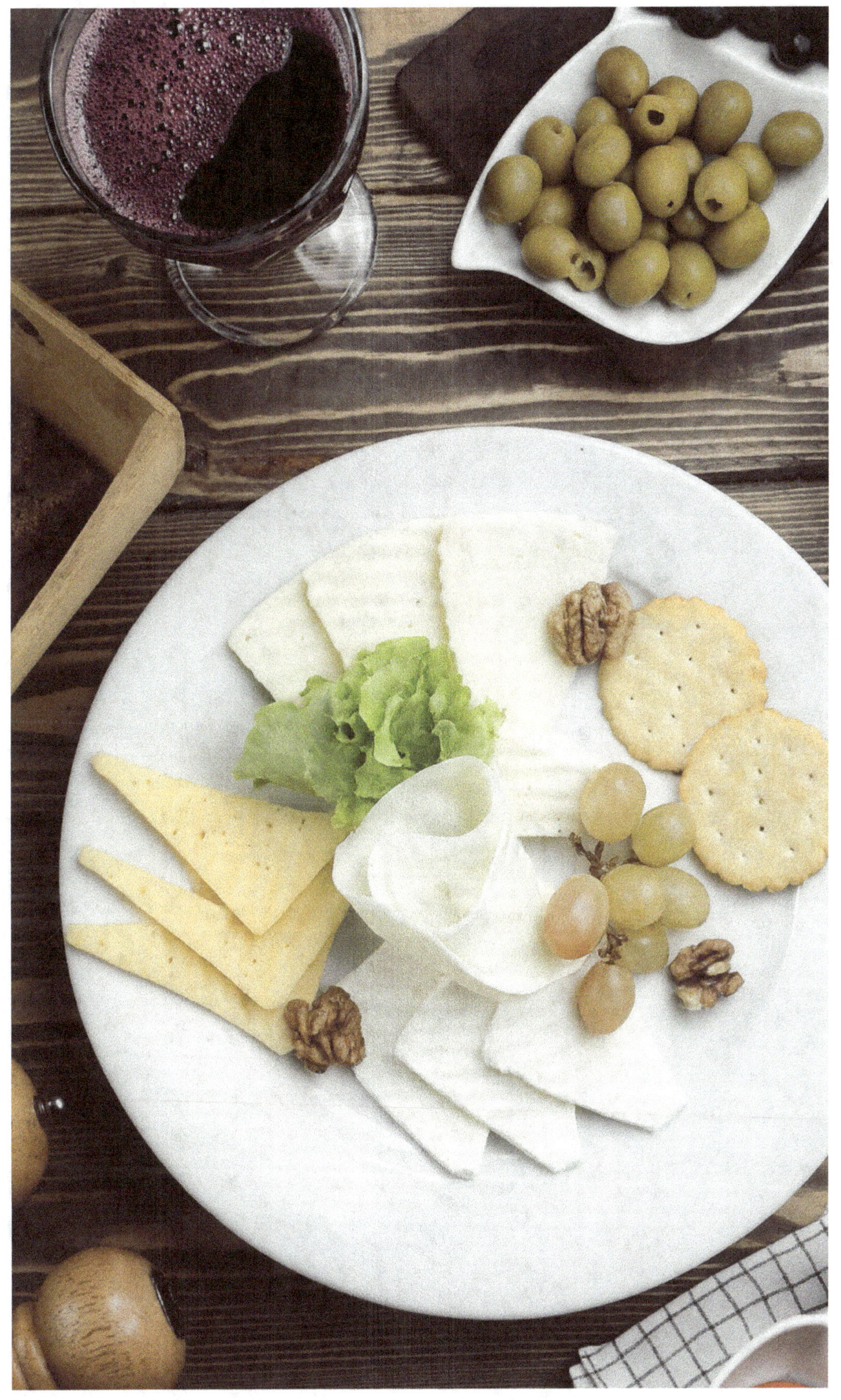

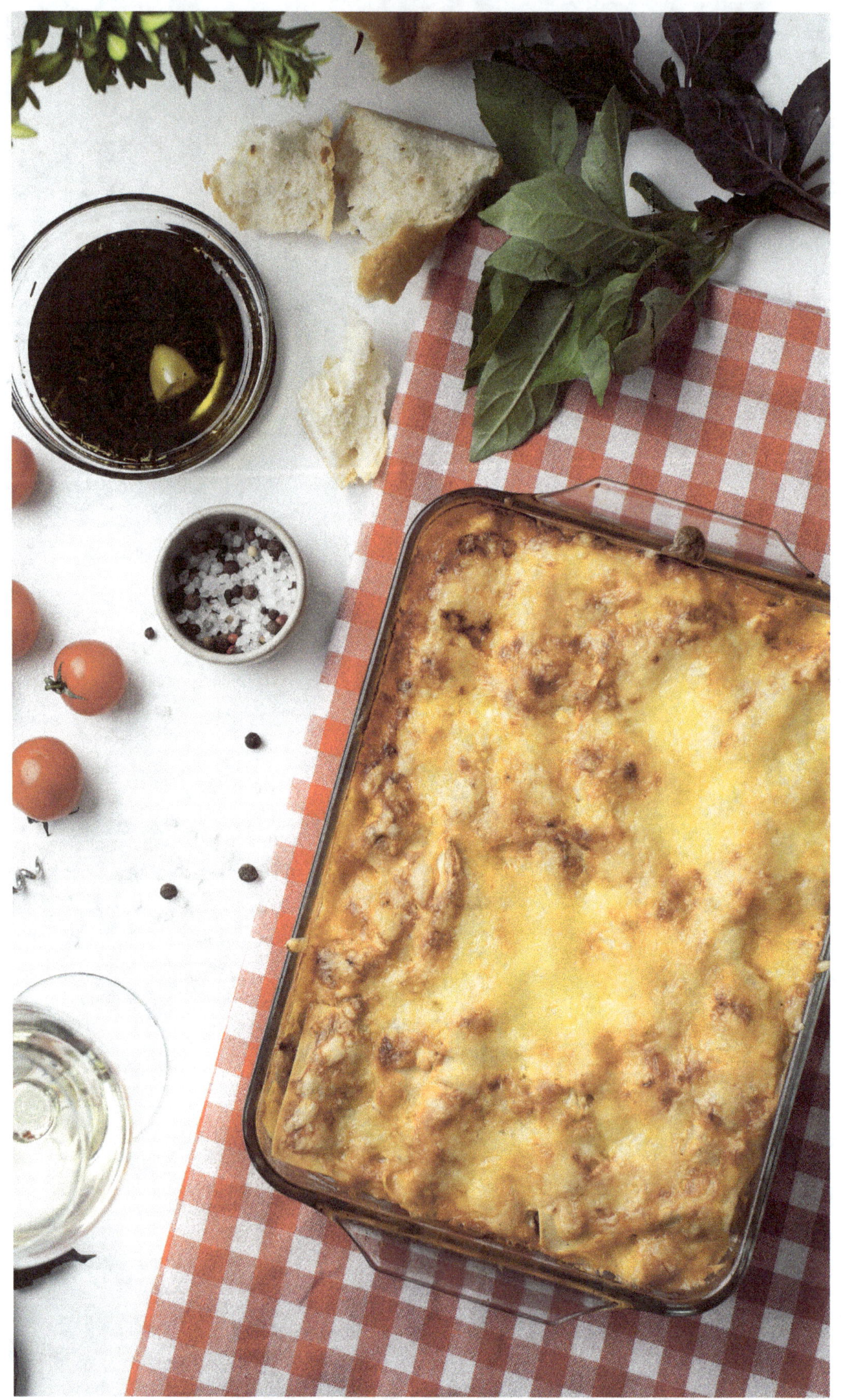

BAKED PASTA CASSEROLE

Spoon Rating: 🍴🍴🍴
Makes: 6 servings
Texture: Soft pasta, melty cheese, hearty sauce
Temperature: Hot
Prep Time: 15 minutes
Calories per serving: ~450–500
Sensory Notes: Familiar, comforting, mild flavors

This casserole is hearty, comforting, and easy to prepare with just a few simple ingredients with lots of leftovers. Using jarred marinara sauce keeps prep minimal, while ground sirloin, chicken, or turkey provides a protein base. Combine with your favorite pasta shape, penne works especially well, and a layer of melty cheese for a satisfying dish that reheats beautifully.

1 lb ground sirloin, ground chicken, or ground turkey

1 jar (24 oz) marinara sauce

12 oz pasta (penne, ziti, or rotini)

2 cups shredded mozzarella cheese

½ cup grated parmesan cheese (optional)

1 tablespoon olive oil

1 teaspoon salt

½ teaspoon garlic powder (optional, mild flavor)

½ teaspoon pepper (optional)

1. Preheat oven to 375°F (190°C). Lightly grease a 9x13-inch casserole dish.
2. Cook pasta in salted water until just al dente. Drain and set aside.
3. Heat olive oil in a large skillet over medium heat. Add ground sirloin, chicken, or turkey, season with salt and mild seasonings, and cook until browned.
4. Stir in the jar of marinara sauce and let simmer for 5 minutes.
5. In a large bowl, mix the cooked pasta with the sauce and meat mixture.
6. Transfer to the casserole dish. Sprinkle mozzarella evenly on top and parmesan if using.
7. Bake for 20–25 minutes, until the cheese is bubbly and lightly golden.
8. Let rest for 5 minutes before serving.

FREEZER BREAKFAST EGG MUFFINS

Spoon Rating: 🥄🥄🥄
Makes: 12 muffins
Texture: Soft, fluffy, lightly chewy
Temperature: Hot
Prep Time: 10 minutes
Calories per serving: ~100–120 per muffin (depends on add-ins)
Sensory Notes: Savory, customizable, satisfying

These little egg muffins are like mini crustless quiches baked in a muffin tin. They're perfect for busy mornings because you can make a big batch, freeze them, and reheat as needed. You can mix and match add-ins depending on what you like or what you have on hand.

10 large eggs

½ cup milk

½ tsp salt

¼ tsp pepper (optional)

½ cup shredded cheese (cheddar, mozzarella, or your favorite)

Optional Add-Ins:

Cooked crumbled bacon
Cooked sausage
Diced tomatoes
Chopped spinach
Bell peppers, diced
Mushrooms, chopped
Chopped green onions

1. Preheat oven to 350°F (175°C). Grease a standard 12-cup muffin tin.
2. In a medium bowl, whisk eggs, milk, salt, and pepper until well combined.
3. Stir in shredded cheese and any add-ins you want to use.
4. Divide the mixture evenly between the muffin cups, filling each about ¾ full.
5. Bake for 20–25 minutes, or until eggs are set and tops are lightly golden.
6. Let muffins cool before removing from the tin. Store in the fridge for up to 4 days or freeze in an airtight bag for up to 2 months. To reheat, microwave for 30–60 seconds.

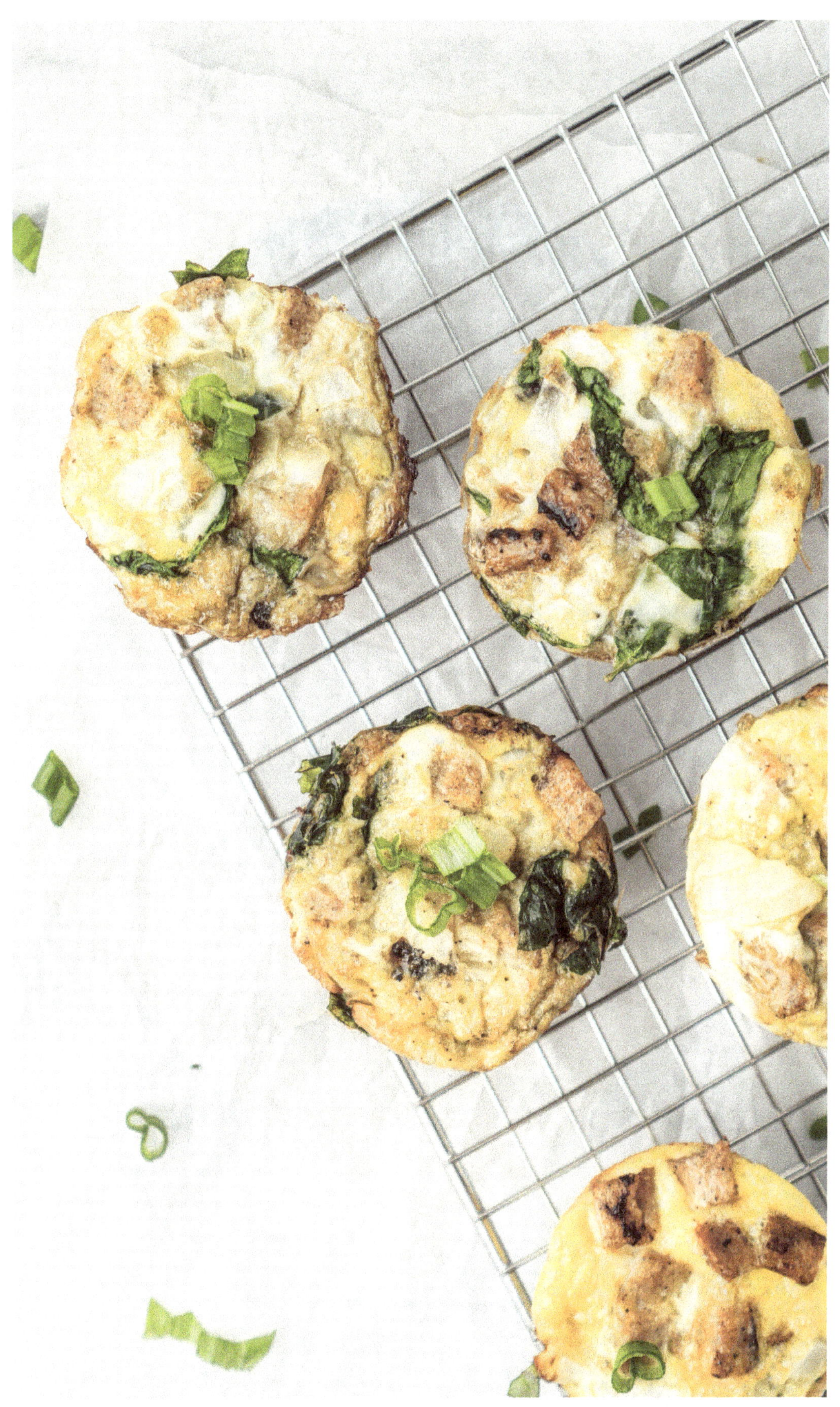

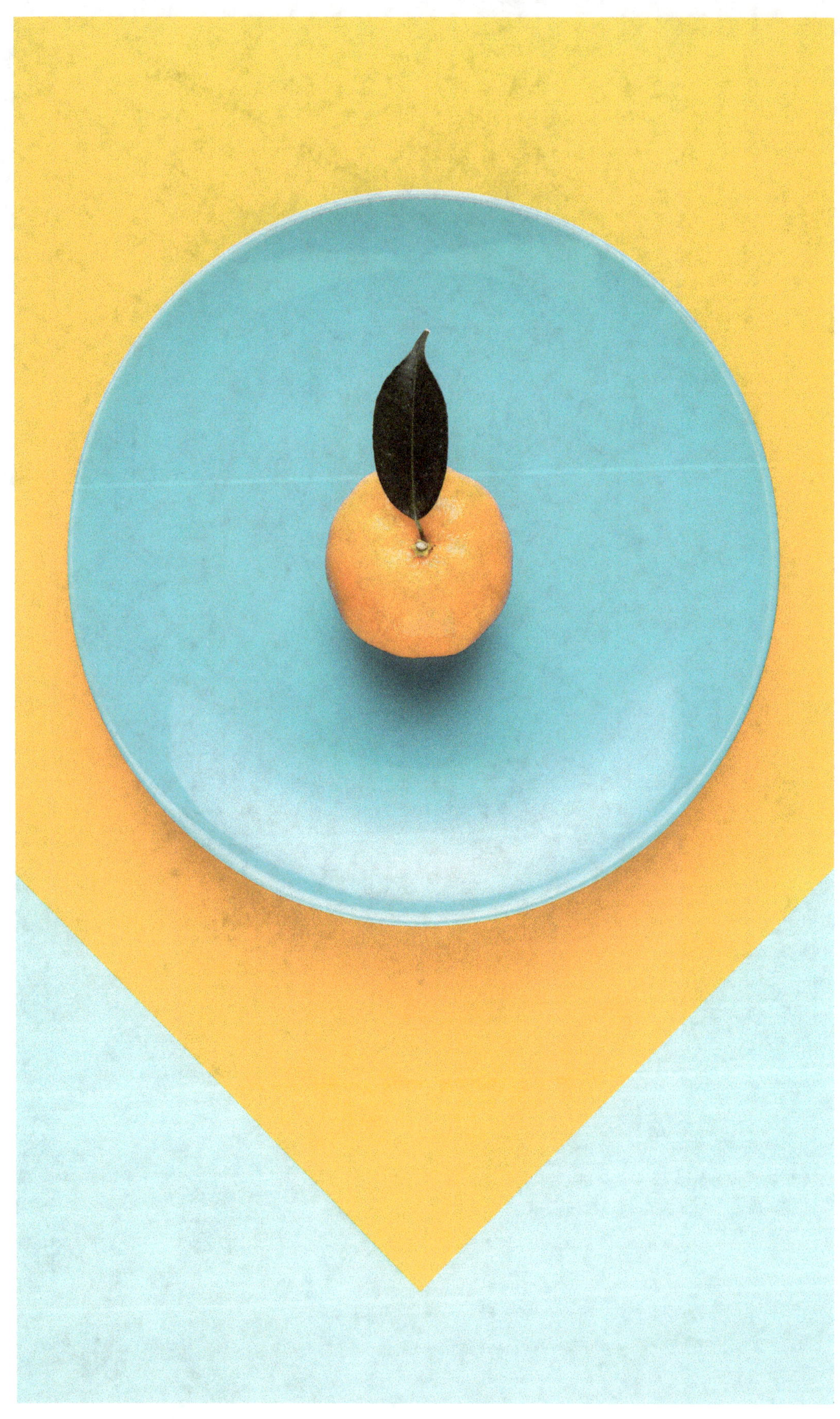

CHAPTER 10: ARFID-FOCUSED SOLUTIONS

Avoidant/Restrictive Food Intake Disorder (ARFID) can make eating feel overwhelming because it often limits the range of safe foods a person feels comfortable with. The goal in this chapter is not to push past those boundaries but to work gently within them. These recipes and tips focus on maximizing nutrition, calories, and comfort while honoring the textures and flavors that feel safe. By leaning on familiar foods, small adjustments can gradually add more nourishment without making meals feel intimidating or unsafe.

One simple way to boost nutrition in safe foods is by adding calorie-dense but nearly tasteless ingredients. For example, a spoonful of coconut oil or MCT oil (a form of medium-chain triglycerides that has almost no flavor) can easily melt into pasta, oatmeal, smoothies, or even mashed potatoes without changing the taste or texture. These invisible boosts can make a big difference for people with ARFID who might struggle to eat larger portions. If this chapter is being used to support a child with ARFID, it's important to consult with their doctor or nutritionist before making changes, so that every adjustment is both safe and supportive. The focus here is on subtle, respectful transformations that keep food feeling safe while giving the body more of what it needs.

CONCENTRATED NUTRITION DRINK

Spoon Rating: ⫶⫶
Makes: 1 serving
Texture: Smooth and creamy
Temperature: Cold
Prep Time: 5 minutes
Calories per serving: ~300–420
Sensory Notes: Creamy banana base, rich vanilla or chocolate flavor, mild and easy to drink

This nutritional drink is extra simple and designed to pack in calories and protein with a very smooth texture. You can choose vanilla or chocolate protein powder depending on your flavor preference, or use a nutritional drink such as Pediasure or Ensure in place of milk. The banana adds creaminess, and the optional MCT oil or coconut oil makes it even more calorie-dense without changing the flavor too much.

1 cup cold whole milk (or non-dairy milk, or nutritional drink)

½ frozen banana

1 scoop vanilla or chocolate protein powder

1 tablespoon honey or maple syrup (optional, for extra sweetness)

1 tablespoon MCT oil or coconut oil (optional, for extra calories)

1. Add all ingredients into a high-speed blender.
2. Blend until completely smooth.
3. Taste and adjust sweetness if needed.
4. Serve cold, or refrigerate for up to 24 hours.

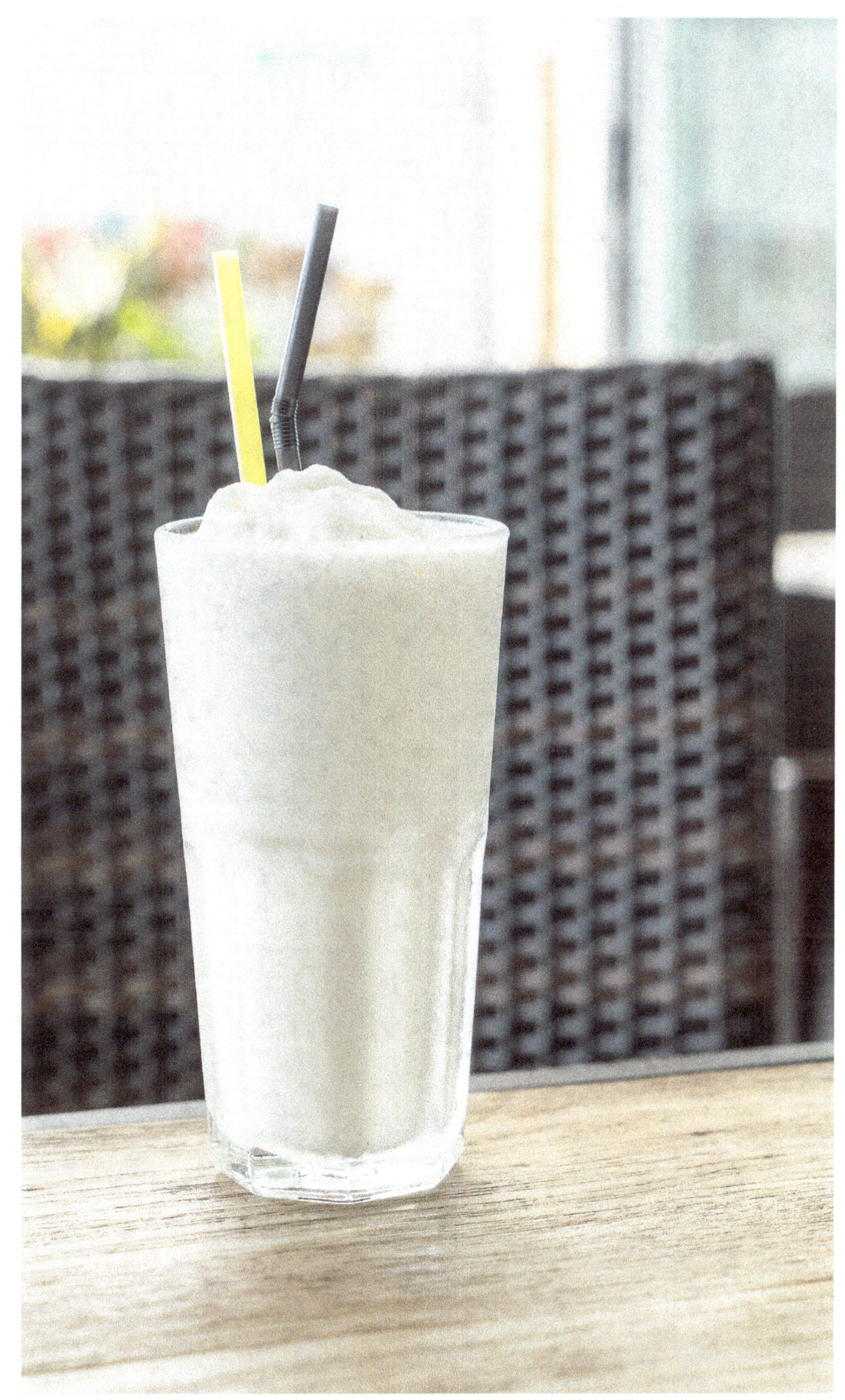

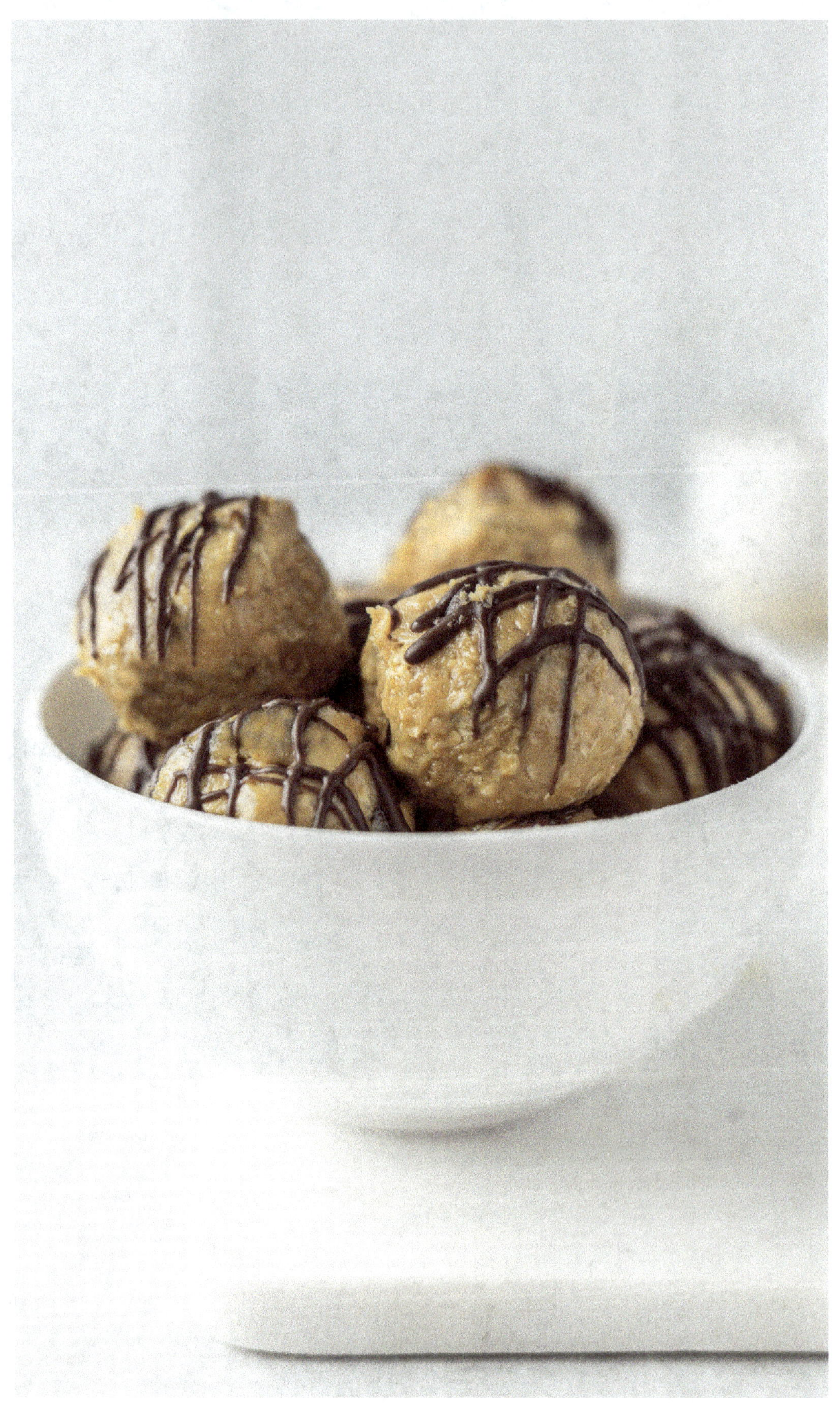

HIGH-ENERGY SNACK BALLS WITH CHOCOLATE SAUCE

Spoon Rating: 🥄🥄🥄
Makes: 12–14 balls
Texture: Soft and chewy inside
Temperature: Cool or room
Prep Time: 10–15 minutes
Calories per serving: ~115 per ball (without sauce)
Sensory Notes: Mild sweetness, nutty and smooth with optional chocolate contrast

These snack balls are soft, simple, and calorie-dense without being overwhelming. The beige-brown color makes them approachable, and the optional chocolate dipping sauce adds comfort without taking away from the mild flavor.

1 cup almond flour

½ cup smooth almond butter (or sunflower butter for nut-free)

¼ cup honey or maple syrup

½ teaspoon vanilla extract

Pinch of salt

For Chocolate Sauce:

½ cup semi-sweet chocolate chips

1 teaspoon coconut oil

1. In a medium bowl, combine almond flour, almond butter, honey, vanilla, and salt. Stir until a soft dough forms.
2. Roll into small bite-sized balls (about 12–14). Place on a parchment-lined plate.
3. For dipping sauce: melt chocolate chips with coconut oil in the microwave in 20-second bursts, stirring until smooth.
4. Serve the snack balls plain or dip lightly into chocolate sauce.
5. Store leftovers in the fridge for up to 5 days.

HIGH-CALORIE CHEESE SAUCE

Spoon Rating: 🍴🍴🍴
Makes: About 2 cups sauce
Texture: Smooth, creamy, melty
Temperature: Hot
Prep Time: 5 minutes
Calories per serving: ~300–350
Sensory Notes: Familiar cheesy flavor, mild, velvety consistency

This sauce is designed to be soft, creamy, and calorie-rich, while still neutral enough for selective eaters. Using whole milk, heavy cream, and butter boosts the calories, while the melted cheese gives a comforting, familiar taste. Can be served over pasta, rice, or as a dipping sauce.

2 tablespoons butter

2 tablespoons all-purpose flour

1 cup whole milk

½ cup heavy cream

2 cups shredded mild cheese (cheddar, mozzarella, or American all work)

½ teaspoon salt (or to taste)

1. In a saucepan over medium heat, melt the butter.
2. Whisk in the flour to make a smooth paste (roux), cooking for about 1 minute.
3. Slowly add the milk and cream, whisking constantly until smooth and slightly thickened (about 3–4 minutes).
4. Stir in the shredded cheese, one handful at a time, until melted and silky.
5. Taste and add salt if needed.
6. Serve immediately over pasta, rice, vegetables, or as a dipping sauce.

CALORIE-DENSE PASTA

Spoon Rating: 🍴🍴🍴
Makes: 4 servings
Texture: Velvety, creamy sauce with tender pasta
Temperature: Hot
Prep Time: 20 minutes
Calories per serving: ~650–800
Sensory Notes: Mild, cheesy, neutral beige color, very smooth and rich

This recipe is designed to be calorie-dense while staying visually neutral, which can be helpful if colorful foods feel overwhelming. It uses familiar, mild flavors with no strong seasoning, just cream, butter, and cheese, making it comforting, filling, and approachable. Use your favorite pasta shape, whether that's penne, rotini, or simple spaghetti.

12 oz pasta (any favorite type)

1 cup heavy cream

4 oz cream cheese, cubed

½ cup grated Parmesan cheese

1 cup shredded mozzarella

2 tablespoons butter

Salt to taste

½ teaspoon pepper (optional)

1. Cook pasta according to package directions. Drain and set aside.
2. In a large saucepan over medium heat, melt the butter. Add heavy cream and let it warm gently.
3. Stir in cream cheese, whisking until smooth.
4. Add Parmesan and mozzarella, stirring until melted and creamy.
5. Season lightly with salt, then add the pasta and stir to coat evenly. Serve warm.

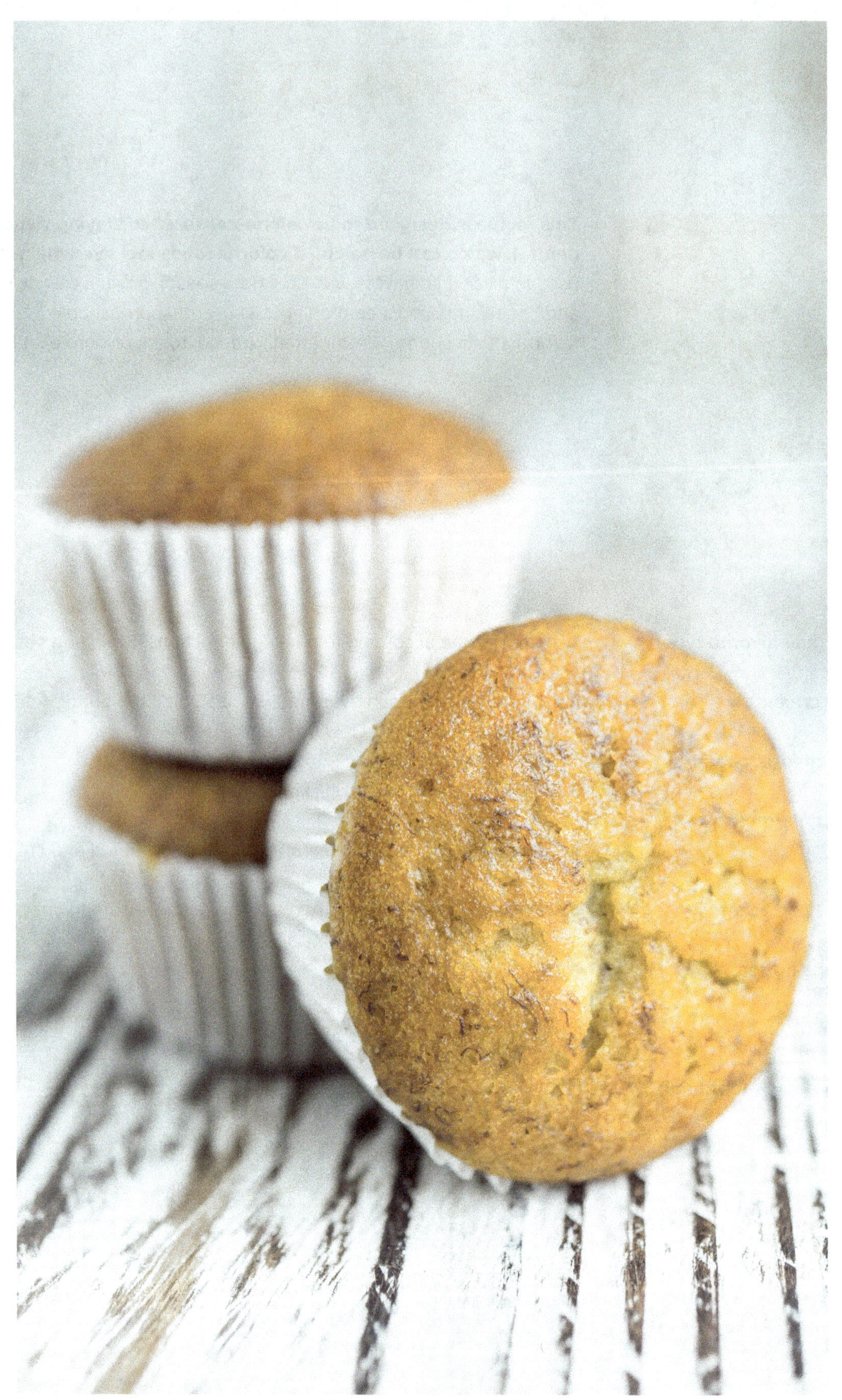

ENERGY-DENSE MUFFINS

Spoon Rating: 🥄🥄🥄🥄
Makes: 12 muffins
Texture: Soft, smooth crumb
Temperature: Warm or room
Prep Time: 10–15 minutes
Calories per serving: ~200–220
Sensory Notes: Mildly sweet, simple, no chunks

These muffins are soft, simple, and calorie-rich without any distracting chunks or textures. They're designed to be neutral in flavor and beige in color, making them approachable for selective eaters. Adding whole milk and a bit of oil makes them especially moist and filling.

1 ½ cups all-purpose flour

½ cup sugar

2 teaspoons baking powder

½ teaspoon salt

2 large eggs

½ cup whole milk

½ cup vegetable oil (or melted butter)

1 teaspoon vanilla extract

1. Preheat oven to 350°F (175°C). Line a 12-cup muffin tin with paper liners.
2. In a medium bowl, whisk together flour, sugar, baking powder, and salt.
3. In a separate bowl, whisk eggs, milk, oil, and vanilla until smooth.
4. Pour the wet ingredients into the dry and mix gently until just combined (don't overmix).
5. Divide the batter evenly among muffin cups, filling about ¾ full.
6. Bake for 18–20 minutes, or until a toothpick inserted in the center comes out clean.
7. Cool slightly before serving.

LIQUID MEAL SOUP

Spoon Rating: 🥄🥄🥄🥄
Makes: 4 servings
Texture: Silky, smooth, drinkable
Temperature: Hot
Prep Time: 25 minutes
Calories per serving: ~280
Sensory Notes: Mild, comforting, soft flavor with no chunks

This soup is mild in flavor, beige-yellow in color, and blends into a creamy liquid that feels more like a warm drink than a chunky meal. It's made with simple, familiar ingredients: potatoes, carrots, and shredded chicken, then blended until smooth.

2 medium potatoes, peeled and diced

2 medium carrots, peeled and chopped

2 cups cooked shredded chicken (use rotisserie or precooked for ease)

4 cups chicken broth (or vegetable broth)

1 small onion, chopped (optional, for more depth)

1 tablespoon olive oil or butter

Salt to taste

1. In a large pot, heat olive oil or butter over medium heat. Add onion (if using) and cook until soft.
2. Add potatoes, carrots, and broth. Bring to a boil, then reduce to a simmer. Cook 15–20 minutes until potatoes and carrots are tender.
3. Add shredded chicken. Simmer for another 5 minutes.
4. Carefully transfer mixture to a high-speed blender and blend until completely smooth.
5. Taste and season with salt as needed.
6. Serve warm in a mug or bowl.

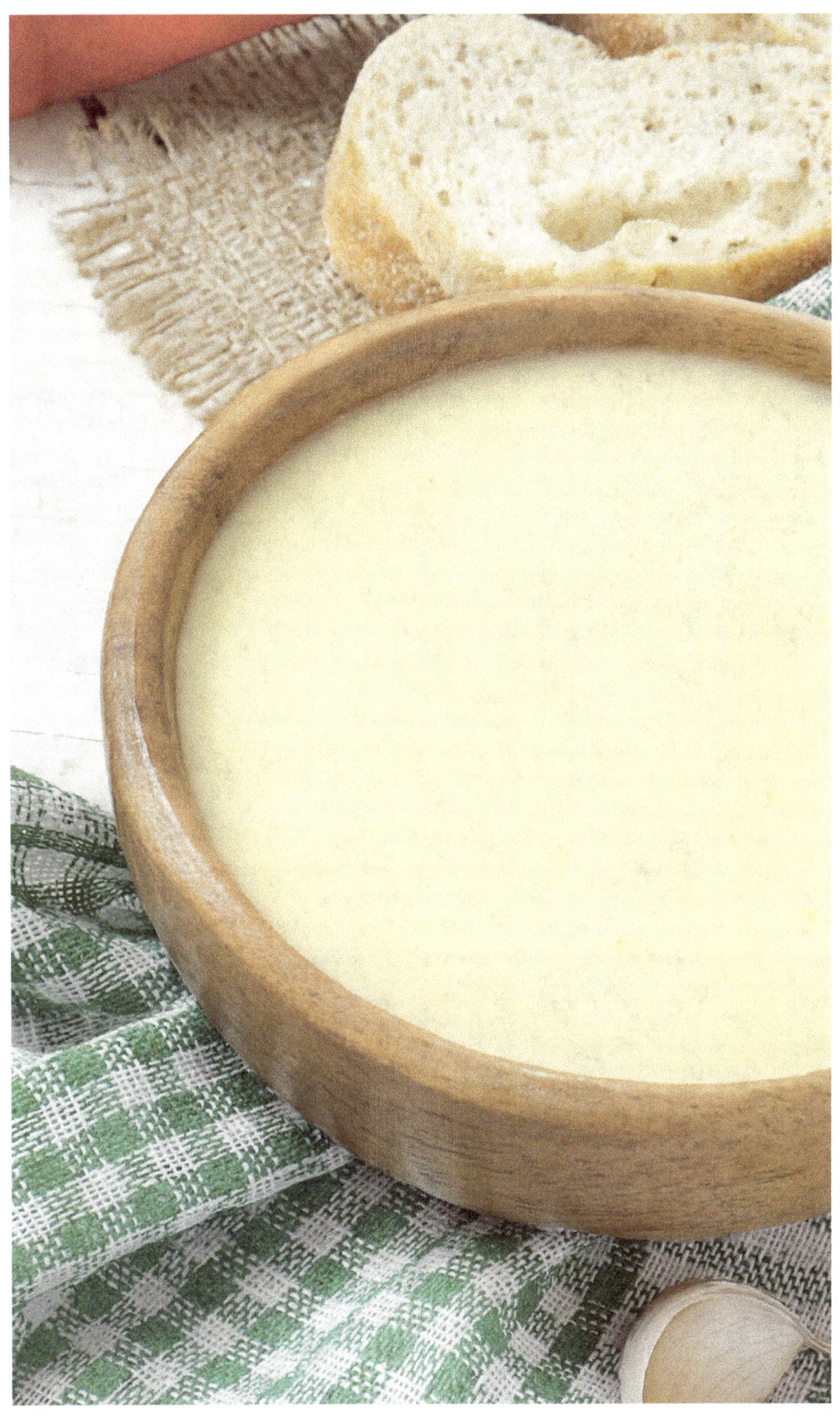

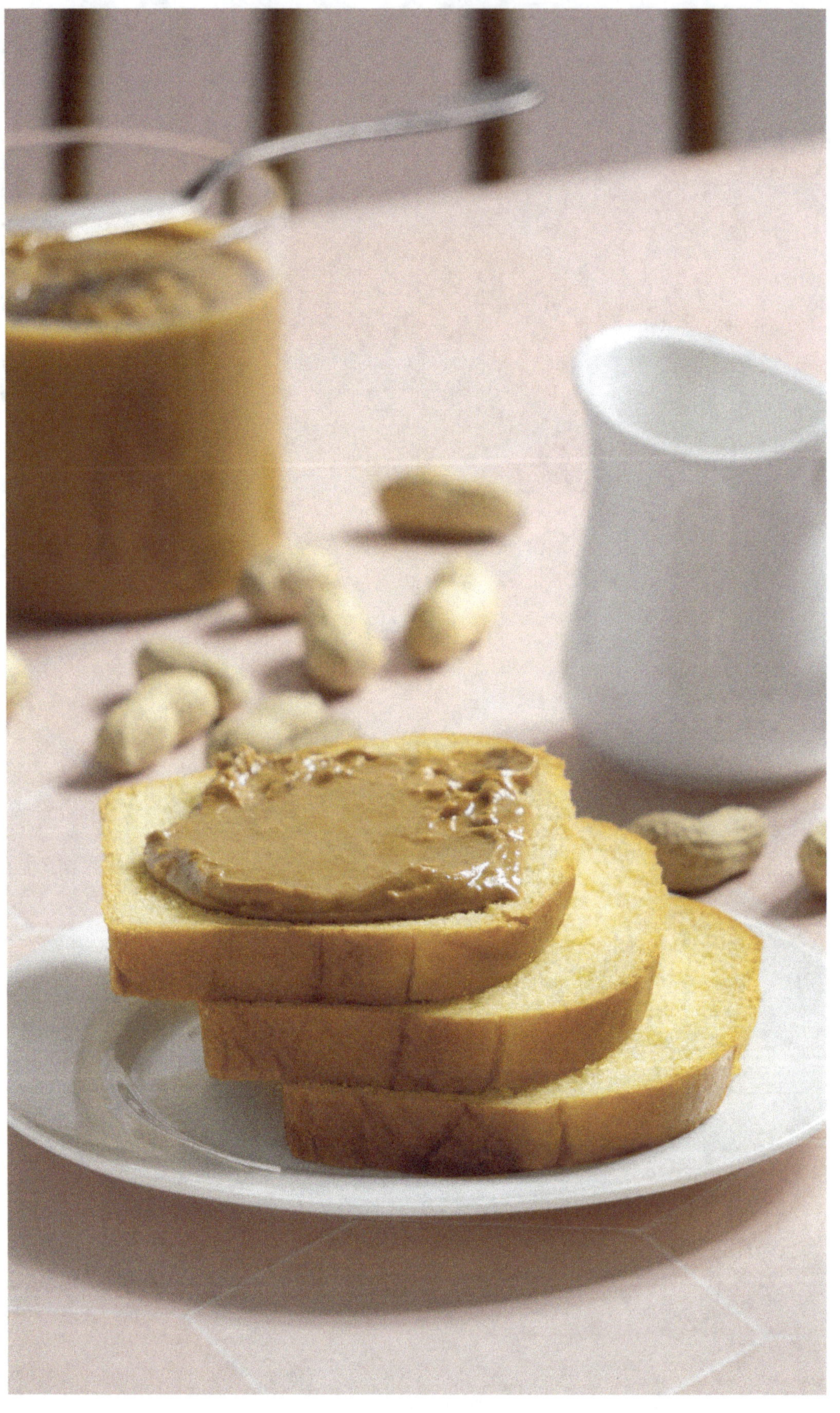

CALORIE-PACKED TOAST

Spoon Rating: 1 spoon
Makes: 1 serving
Texture: Soft with light crunch if toasted
Temperature: Warm or room
Prep Time: 10–15 minutes
Calories per serving: ~300–350
Sensory Notes: Familiar nutty flavor, mild, creamy

This toast is a simple way to add extra calories and healthy fats without changing the texture or overwhelming the flavor. MCT oil (medium-chain triglycerides, often made from coconut oil) has almost no taste, making it a great way to boost energy intake. If preparing for a child, always check with their doctor or nutritionist before adding oils or supplements.

1–2 slices of soft white bread (or your favorite bread)

2 tablespoons creamy peanut butter

1 teaspoon MCT oil (start with less if needed, since it can be rich)

Honey or banana slices (optional for extra calories and sweetness)

1. Toast the bread lightly (or leave untoasted if preferred for texture).
2. In a small bowl, mix the peanut butter and MCT oil until smooth.
3. Spread the mixture evenly over the bread.
4. Top with honey or banana slices if desired.

PROTEIN-PACKED PANCAKES

Spoon Rating: 🍴🍴🍴
Makes: About 6 small pancakes
Texture: Soft, fluffy, slightly dense
Temperature: Warm
Prep Time: 5 minutes
Calories per serving: ~120–150 (varies with protein powder)
Sensory Notes: Mild flavor, soft chew, lightly sweet

These pancakes are a filling, high-energy option that delivers extra protein without losing the comfort of a classic breakfast food. They're beige in color and mildly flavored, so they won't feel overwhelming.

1 cup all-purpose flour

1 scoop vanilla or chocolate protein powder (about 25–30g)

1 tablespoon sugar (optional)

2 teaspoons baking powder

Pinch of salt

1 cup milk (dairy or non-dairy)

1 large egg

2 tablespoons melted butter or coconut oil (plus extra for frying)

1. In a mixing bowl, whisk together flour, protein powder, sugar, baking powder, and salt.
2. In another bowl, whisk milk, egg, and melted butter or oil.
3. Combine wet and dry ingredients, stirring gently until just combined (don't overmix). Batter should be slightly thick.
4. Heat a nonstick skillet or griddle over medium-low heat and lightly coat with butter or oil.
5. Pour ¼ cup batter for each pancake. Cook until bubbles form on the surface (about 2 minutes), then flip and cook until golden brown (1–2 minutes more).
6. Serve warm with syrup, nut butter, or a drizzle of honey for extra calories.

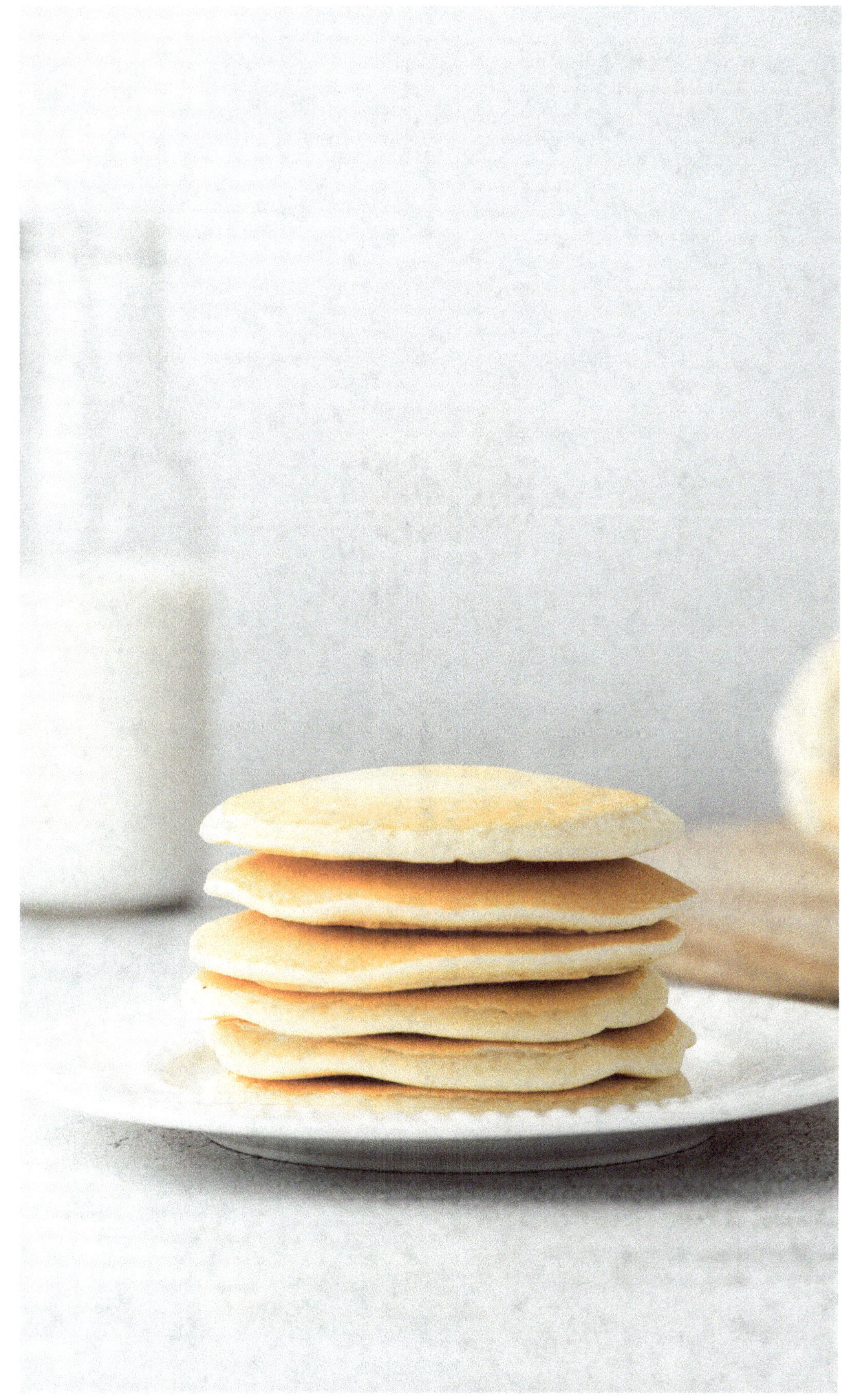

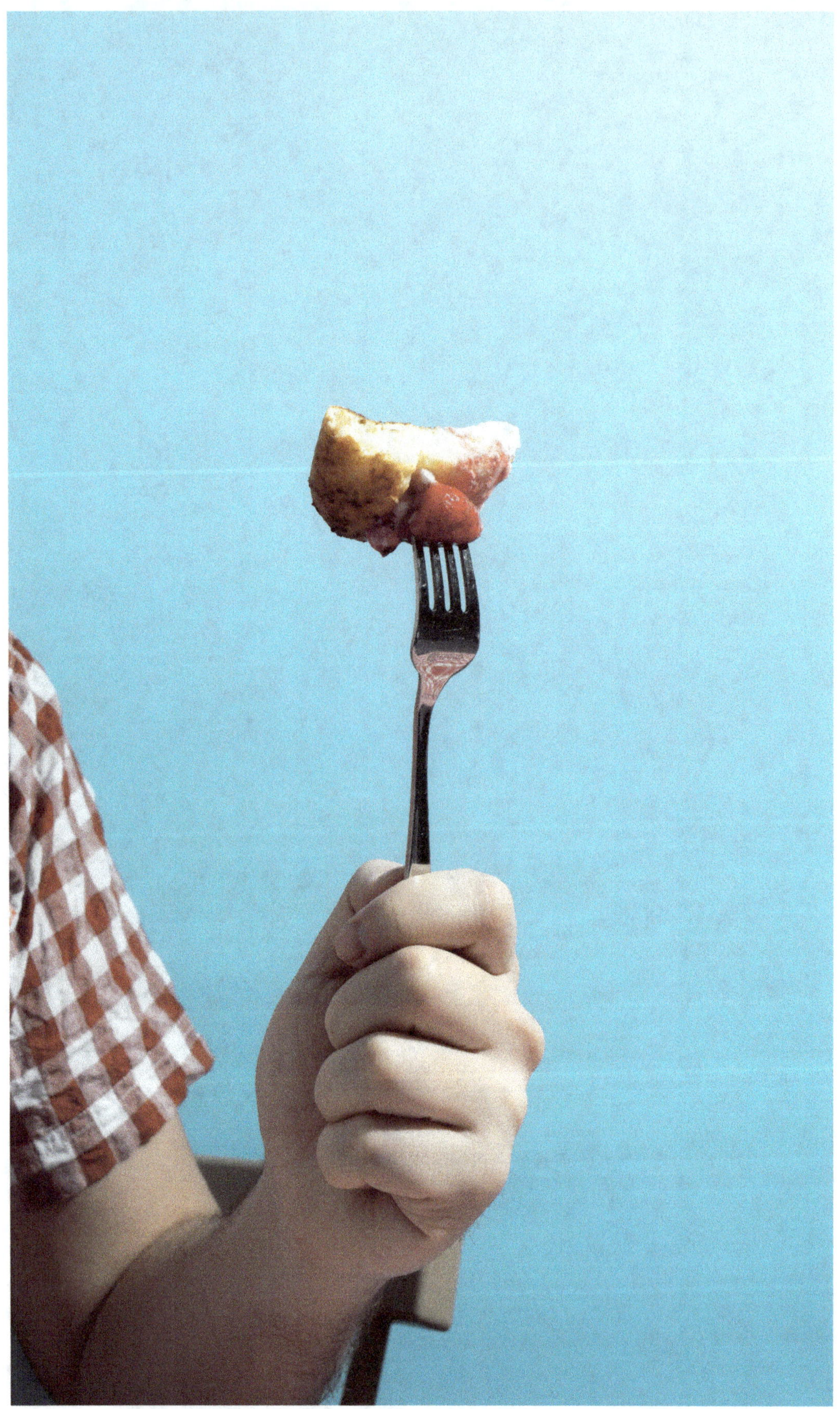

CHAPTER 11: FOOD CHAINING ADVENTURES

Food chaining is a gentle, step-by-step approach to expanding what someone is willing to eat. The idea is simple: you start with a food that feels safe and familiar, then slowly introduce a new food that shares a similar taste, texture, or appearance. Over time, these small, low-stress steps create a bridge from comfort foods to new, more varied options. This approach is often used for individuals with ARFID (Avoidant/Restrictive Food Intake Disorder) or sensory sensitivities, but it can be just as useful for picky eaters of any age who want to feel more comfortable trying new things.

In the following pages, you'll see examples of food chaining in action. Each recipe in this book can become a starting point for gentle experimentation, whether it's one single sprinkle to ice cream, adjusting the size of chocolate chips in cookies, or swapping one cheese for another. The key is gradual change, where familiar flavors remain present and safe while new foods are carefully layered in. Think of it as building a bridge, one small step at a time, where every link connects to what you already know and enjoy. This makes mealtime less overwhelming and gives you more confidence to explore.

FOOD CHAINING IDEAS

1. Scrambled Eggs (page 78) → Scrambled Eggs with a Pinch of Shredded Cheese
2. Scrambled Eggs (page 78) → Eggs with ½ teaspoon of Crumbled Bacon
3. Chicken Tenders (page 38) → Chicken Tenders with Cornflakes Mixed into Breadcrumbs
4. Chicken Nuggets (page 41) → Chicken Nuggets with Panko Mixed into Breadcrumbs
5. Plain Chicken Patty (page 50) → Patty with ¼ teaspoon of Ground Pepper
6. Pasta with Butter (page 60) → Pasta with ½ teaspoon of Olive Oil
7. Pasta with Butter (page 60) → Pasta with a ½ teaspoon of Fresh Finely Cut Herbs
8. Pasta with Butter (page 60) → Pasta with a Drop of Alfredo Sauce
9. White Rice (page 63) → Rice with ½ teaspoon of Brown Rice
10. White Rice (page 63) → Rice with ½ teaspoon of Garlic Salt
11. Rice Cake → Rice Cake with One Sunflower Seed Pressed In
12. Rice Cake → Rice Cake with Thin Layer of Chocolate Spread
13. French Fries with Ketchup → French Fries with Ketchup with a Drop of Vinegar
14. Hamburger (page 59) → Hamburger with One Small Piece of Lettuce
15. Cheese Pizza → Cheese Pizza with a Dash of Oregano
16. Cheese Pizza → Cheese Pizza with One Corner Dipped In Ranch Dressing
17. Grilled Cheese (page 69) → Grilled Cheese with Paper-Thin Tomato
18. Grilled Cheese (page 69) → Grilled Cheese with Cheese Brand Slightly Different
19. White Bread Sandwich → Sandwich with Crust Edge Left On
20. Plain Bagel → Bagel with a Few Sesame Seeds
21. Plain Tortilla → Tortilla with One Dot of Smooth Salsa Spread Thin
22. Plain Tortilla with Cheese → Tortilla with Different Brand Cheese Mixed with Favorite Cheese
23. Safe Soup → Soup with One Drop from a Different Soup
24. Mashed Potatoes (page 66) → Mashed Potatoes with a ½ Cup Heavy Cream
25. Mashed Potatoes (page 66) → Mashed Potatoes with a Few Shreds of Mild White Cheese

26 Mashed Potatoes (page 66) → Mashed Potatoes with ½ teaspoon of Parmesan Cheese

27 Toast → Toast with Barely-There Cinnamon

28 Toast → Toast with Invisible Brush of Olive Oil Under Butter

29 Plain Crackers → Crackers with the Thinnest Smear of Cream Cheese

30 Plain Crackers → Crackers with a Crumb-Sized Piece of Ham or Turkey

31 Plain Crackers → Crackers with One Grain of Sea Salt

32 Plain Crackers → Crackers with Dust of Powdered Cheese

33 Plain Oatmeal → Oatmeal with ½ teaspoon of Brown Sugar Crystal

34 Plain Oatmeal → Oatmeal with ½ teaspoon of Honey

35 Plain Yogurt → Yogurt with Small Drizzle of Honey

36 Plain Yogurt → Yogurt with One Small Slice of Banana Blended In

37 Vanilla Smoothie (page 22) → Smoothie with a Few Blueberries Finely Blended

38 Vanilla Pudding → Pudding with One Sprinkle of Cinnamon Sugar

39 Vanilla Ice Cream → Vanilla Ice Cream with a Single Chocolate Sprinkle on Top

40 Vanilla Ice Cream → Ice Cream with Drizzle of Honey

41 Safe Muffin (page 153) → Safe Muffin with a Dash of Sugar on Top

42 Safe Muffin (page 153) → Safe Muffin with a Thin Layer of Chocolate Spread on Top

43 Safe Cookie → Cookie with Tiny Piece of Raisen

44 Chocolate Chip Cookies (page 74) → Chocolate Chip Cookies with Hand Cut Chocolate Chunks

45 Apple Slice → Apple Slice Brushed with Lemon Juice

46 Smooth Peanut Butter → Peanut Butter with a Dash of Sprinkles

47 Plain Popcorn → Popcorn with a Few Chocolate Chips Mixed In

48 Plain Milk → Milk with a Tiny Drop of Vanilla Extract

49 Safe Cereal → Cereal with ½ Cup Different Cereal Mixed In

50 Plain Pancake (page 73) → Pancake with One Drip of Honey Spread Out

INDEX

A

All-purpose flour – 38, 41, 46, 50, 51, 67, 70, 73, 74, 101, 109, 118, 121, 122, 125, 126, 141, 150, 153, 158
Almond butter – 31, 149
Almond flour – 149
Apple – 34, 82, 89, 138
Apple juice – 33
Avocado – 85, 130

B

Baking powder – 73, 121, 122, 125, 153, 158
Baking soda – 74, 109, 121, 126
Banana – 22, 25, 26, 29, 31, 110, 146, 157
Barbecue sauce – 49, 54
Bay leaf – 42
Beef – 59, 119, 130, 137, 141
Beef broth – 137
Bell pepper – 102, 134, 138, 142
Blueberries – 33, 82
Bread – 64, 67, 69, 85, 89, 138, 157
Breadcrumbs – 38, 41, 46, 50, 51, 70, 101, 119, 141
Broccoli – 102, 134
Brown sugar – 74, 109, 126
Butter – 60, 64, 66, 67, 69, 70, 73, 81, 97, 114, 135, 150, 151, 158
Butternut squash – 114

C

Carrots – 86, 90, 118, 137, 138, 154
Cashews – 102
Cauliflower – 117
Chamomile tea – 29
Cheddar cheese – 69, 70, 81, 87, 105, 114, 130, 133, 135, 138, 142, 150, 151
Chicken breast – 38, 41, 42, 45, 49, 53, 102, 134
Chicken broth – 42, 49, 97, 135, 154
Chicken drumsticks – 46
Chicken thighs – 49, 53
Chicken wings – 54
Chickpeas – 98
Chocolate chips – 74, 109, 121, 125, 126, 149
Cocoa powder – 25, 121, 125
Coconut (shredded) – 101
Coconut oil – 67, 73, 122, 146, 149, 158
Coconut water – 30, 33, 34
Cornstarch – 74
Cream cheese – 135, 151
Cucumber – 34, 105

E

Eggs – 38, 41, 46, 50, 51, 67, 78, 101, 117, 119, 121, 122, 125, 126, 142, 153, 158

F

Flour (see All-purpose flour)

G

Garlic – 97, 102, 135
Garlic powder – 38, 41, 45, 46, 49, 50, 51, 53, 94, 114, 117, 118, 119, 134, 141
Ginger – 42
Grapes (green) – 34
Greek yogurt – 22, 25, 29, 31, 87, 105, 107
Ground beef/sirloin – 59, 119, 130, 141
Ground chicken – 50, 51, 119, 141
Ground turkey – 50, 51, 119, 141

H

Heavy cream – 150, 151
Honey – 22, 25, 26, 29, 30, 31, 82, 107, 122, 126, 146, 149, 157
Hummus – 98

I

Ice cubes – 22, 25, 26
Italian seasoning – 135, 137

L

Lemon juice – 34, 85, 98, 105
Lemon/lime – 34
Lettuce – 133

M

Mango – 30, 33
Maple syrup – 22, 25, 26, 29, 31, 107, 146
Marinara sauce – 118, 119, 141
Mayonnaise – 105, 133
MCT oil – 146, 157
Milk – 22, 25, 26, 66, 73, 78, 114, 121, 122, 135, 142, 146, 150, 151, 153, 158
Mozzarella cheese – 70, 117, 130, 135, 141, 150, 151
Mustard – 133

O

Oats (rolled) – 109
Olive oil – 45, 87, 94, 97, 98, 102, 118, 134, 135, 137, 141, 154
Onion – 97, 102, 119, 137, 154
Orange juice – 33

P

Panko breadcrumbs – 46
Paprika – 38, 41, 46, 53, 94
Parmesan cheese – 51,

70, 118, 135, 151
Pasta – 60, 105, 118, 135, 141, 151
Peaches – 26, 30, 33
Peanut butter – 25, 31, 157
Pepper – 38, 41, 45, 46, 49, 50, 51, 53, 59, 60, 66, 70, 94, 105, 134, 135, 137, 141, 142, 151
Pineapple – 29, 34
Pita bread – 98, 106
Pomegranate juice – 33
Potatoes – 66, 87, 94, 137, 154
Protein powder – 31, 146, 158
Pumpkin puree – 126

R
Rice – 63, 86, 102
Rice cakes – 162

S
Shrimp – 101
Sour cream – 81, 130
Soy sauce – 102
Spinach – 34, 118
Strawberries – 33
Sugar – 64, 73, 74, 97, 106, 109, 121, 122, 125, 126, 153, 158
Sweet potato puree – 122, 125, 126

T
Tahini – 98
Teriyaki sauce – 86, 102
Thyme – 137
Tomatoes – 97, 105, 133
Tortilla chips – 130
Tortillas – 81, 133
Tuna – 86
Turkey (deli) – 133

V
Vanilla extract – 22, 67, 73, 74, 110, 121, 122, 125, 126, 146, 149, 153
Vegetable broth – 97, 135, 154

W
Water – 30, 34, 42, 49, 60, 63, 78, 82, 98, 137
Watermelon – 33
White sugar (see Sugar)

Y
Yogurt (see Greek yogurt) – 82, 107

Z
Zucchini – 118, 119, 121, 125, 134

ABOUT THE AUTHOR

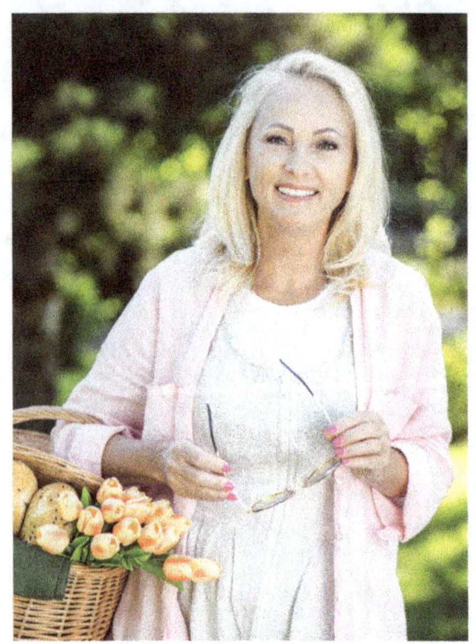

Mary Wojcik knows what it feels like to be called a "picky eater." Now a mother to neurodivergent children with their own unique food needs, she understands firsthand how stressful mealtimes can be and how deeply meaningful it is when food feels safe, nourishing, and full of love. Drawing on her own experiences, Mary creates recipes that are simple, sensory-friendly, and full of compassion. *The Neurodivergent Cookbook* reflects her belief that food should never be a source of shame, but full of comfort and connection.

www.ingramcontent.com/pod-product-compliance
Lightning Source LLC
Chambersburg PA
CBHW080401190726
48411CB00024B/247

9781971159003